The Blood Sugar
Freedom Formula

The Blood Sugar Freedom Formula
Type 1 Diabetes, Simplified

Matt Vande Vegte

Published by Game Changer Publishing

Paperback ISBN: 978-1-964811-88-8
Hardcover ISBN: 978-1-964811-91-8
Digital: ISBN: 978-1-964811-92-5

Medical Disclaimer:
The information provided in this book is for general informational purposes only and is not intended as medical advice. While the author has taken care to ensure the accuracy of the information presented, this book is not a substitute for professional medical advice, diagnosis, or treatment. Always seek the guidance of your physician or other qualified healthcare provider with any questions you may have regarding a medical condition or treatment. Never disregard professional medical advice or delay in seeking it because of something you have read in this book. The author and publisher disclaim any liability for any adverse effects resulting directly or indirectly from the use of the information contained in this book.

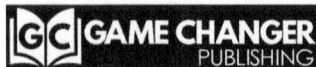

GC | GAME CHANGER PUBLISHING
www.GameChangerPublishing.com

DEDICATION

This book is a tribute to the T1D Warriors—and the caregivers of T1D Warriors—who refuse to be defined by their condition, who greet each day as an opportunity to rewrite the rules of what's possible while living life to the fullest.

To those who understand that true diabetes management is an art form, blending science with intuition to transform challenges into triumphs.

To those who realize there has to be a better way forward with this disease— not just through healthy blood sugars, but also with a happy quality of life and peace of mind.

For the warriors who refuse to be spectators in their own lives, who embrace the complexities of T1D not as obstacles, but as catalysts for growth and self-discovery...

May this book be your compass in navigating the intricate landscape of diabetes, your source of strength in moments of doubt, and your reminder that you are part of a community of resilient fighters.

To every T1D striving for more than just good numbers—for a life rich with adventure, purpose, and joy.

This is your call to action. You now have the tools to answer it.

—

Also to my incredible family for their love, support, and patience as I fought tooth and nail for stability and predictability in my own type 1 diabetes journey. You're the reason I'm still here today and I couldn't have done any of this without you.

Read This First

Just to say thanks for buying and reading my book, and to ensure your success with the methods shared throughout, I would like to give you a free gift, no strings attached!

Scan the QR Code Here:

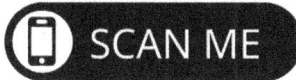

The Blood Sugar Freedom Formula

Type 1 Diabetes, Simplified

Matt Vande Vegte

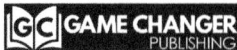

GC GAME CHANGER
PUBLISHING

www.GameChangerPublishing.com

Foreword

In the world of type 1 diabetes (T1D) management, Matt is a true pioneer. His dedication and innovative approach have transformed the lives of countless individuals, myself included, helping us not just manage our condition, but truly master it. As an Ironman competitor, world traveler, and diabetes management expert, Matt offers a wealth of knowledge through his weekly group calls, monthly masterclasses, social media presence, and personalized coaching sessions.

My own T1D journey began with my diagnosis in 1989. For decades, I grappled with the challenges familiar to many: avoiding overeating to correct lows, timing pre-bolus doses correctly, maintaining regular blood sugar checks, and accurately counting carbs. It wasn't until I discovered Matt's work online and later joined his Diabetes in Action program that I experienced a profound shift in my approach to diabetes management.

With Matt's guidance, I set ambitious goals: an A1C below 6% and a time in range above 80%. These targets seemed daunting, but through Matt's methods—including personalized blood sugar formulas and advanced insulin management techniques—I achieved what once seemed impossible. For the first time in over 34 years, I reached 100% time in range and lowered my A1C to 5.5%. These milestones filled me with an overwhelming sense of accomplishment and renewed hope for my future.

When Matt invited me to become an Assistant Coach for the Warrior's Tribe+ community, I knew I had found my calling. The opportunity to help others achieve similar transformations in their health and quality of life was irresistible.

In this book, Matt shares the techniques that revolutionized my approach to diabetes, nutrition, activity, and insulin management. His clear, step-by-step strategies are designed to help you achieve exceptional blood sugar control without constant highs and lows or unnecessary restrictions. By following his approach, you can aim for 90% or more time in range and better A1C results than traditional methods typically yield.

As you read on, you'll discover how to use Matt's formulas and timelines to take control of your blood sugars. By applying these proven techniques, you'll find that diabetes becomes a manageable aspect of your life rather than a constant struggle. I encourage you to join our community, implement these strategies, and prepare for significant positive changes in your life.

Here's to your success and a future filled with possibilities.

Sincerely,

–Trisha Rumple

Assistant Coach, Warrior's Tribe+

Diabetes in Action Graduate

Warrior's Inner Circle Graduate

Century Club Award Winner

Table of Contents

INTRODUCTION

What if there were a way to have blood sugar levels so well controlled that you were able to live your life freely, without worry, and feel "normal" again? While there may not be a cure yet, thousands of type 1 diabetics are experiencing what doctors have told us in the past was impossible: *thriving with type 1 diabetes.* With blood sugars so close to perfection, they're able to live their best lives with fun foods, spontaneous activities, and peace of mind. It's caused a bit of a renegade movement in the diabetes community, so much so that this book was written by popular demand as a plea to get this information out to the rest of the world because of how powerful the concepts you're about to read are. Revolutionary new methods for mastering blood sugars—not through restriction or complicated "rules"—but through a deeper understanding that brings true *freedom* from the shackles of diabetes.

As you read this introduction, you're probably wondering who I am, so let me introduce myself. My name is Matt Vande Vegte, and I'm happy to tell you that I'm *not* a doctor. Why am I happy about that? Well, while I'm grateful for doctors, endocrinologists, dietitians, and the rest of the medical professionals (especially because literally everyone in my family, including my wife, works in the medical field), I was tragically let down by my medical team when it came to my type 1 diabetes care. After speaking with thousands of other type 1s like me over the years as a T1D coach, I've heard far too many similar stories of doctors, endos, dietitians, and so on who just don't get it. Either they're ignorant of what the day-to-day realities of type 1 diabetes look like and make general recommendations from their outdated books that just don't translate to our unique situations, or they just don't have the time or dedication to help me get to my *best*. Their main focus seems to be on just surviving type 1 diabetes (whereas I'd like to focus on *thriving*). So, I sought out a better option—my own path forward as a "renegade."

Now, if your doctor, dietitian, endocrinologist, PA, nurse, diabetes educator, or anyone else from your medical team recommended this book to you… You have one of the good ones. One that is open to what's innovative and new. A medical team member who has held onto their curiosity and strives to improve and seek out the best for their patients. They are few and far between; do not let them go. Many, like myself, are not so lucky and must carve out their own path forward without outside help.

As a renegade, I followed my curiosity and studied to become a certified master fitness trainer and nutritionist to find solutions to erratic blood sugar. I connected with top researchers and diabetes specialists around the world to get answers to the nuances in blood sugar swings that I experienced in my own life. But it wasn't until I nearly died from an urgent low blood sugar crisis in a foreign country (while there by myself) that my curiosity turned into an obsession. I felt a need to identify the perfect blood sugar formula so I could live my life on my terms without diabetes getting in the way ever again. After that near-death experience, my mental health suffered dramatic shifts, and I was even diagnosed with severe anxiety and panic disorder, PTSD, and suicidal ideation. My new mental burden forced me into a *do-or-die* moment, where I truly felt that if I didn't find a solution to my blood sugar issues, I might as well die trying. It put me in a dark place, but I can say now that I'm grateful for it in the end. As you may have figured out, I didn't die, which means that, yes, I did find a solution.

In this book, I look forward to sharing with you the consolidated and fine-tuned solution that I've been using for many years, one that my type 1 diabetes (T1D) clients around the world have been using as well not only to *fix* blood sugar but to do so while living their lives to the absolute fullest. The creation of this book came as a request from my clients after they shared their results from my coaching program with their medical teams and were met with shock, joy, and curiosity. I've come to see that although most doctors and endocrinologists *want* to help, they either don't know how or just don't have the time. My clients demanded that I "spill the secrets" to the world because of the life-changing potential of these counterintuitive new methods. Finally, after years of ideation, iteration, and implementation, we have the results from this new diabetes management strategy to back up our findings, and I've spent the last two years simplifying and consolidating the concepts into the pages you hold within your hands. It's my goal to give you everything you need to dramatically change your life, your perspective, and your outcome with insulin-dependent diabetes.

As a type 1 diabetic myself, I know that a lot of resources, funding, and attention may get diverted to other types of diabetes while we get left to figure out our own insulin-to-carb ratios in the dark, so I want to be clear who this book is for, and conversely, who it is not for.

If you're someone who takes insulin to survive (or loves someone who does), this book is for you. You're likely the kind of person who refuses to settle for anything less than what is best for your own health. You're on a mission to identify the root cause of your blood sugar issues and find lasting solutions, not just slap on Band-Aid fixes and restrictive diets while hoping for the best. You like the idea of precision control over blood sugar that will enable you to enjoy more flexibility with food choices, activity levels, and even spontaneity with more "normalcy" in life. If you're anything like me, you know that a deeper understanding of why things work often yields more peace of mind and confidence in diabetes management (with fewer mystery blood sugar swings).

If you recognize that no one is coming to save us, this book was written for you, and it's time we take responsibility for our own diabetes (even though it wasn't our fault). This book will help you to excel as long as you're the kind of person who takes action and refuses to back down when things get hard. This book will challenge you, but if you're anything like me, it will unlock your "renegade warrior" side, and you'll join the ranks of the thousands of others just like us who *think differently* about diabetes management in order to get the most out of life. Finally, this book is for you if you *know* that life can get better and are willing to *commit* to yourself to see this through and be disciplined enough to read—and take action on—every page in this book.

Once you finish this book, there's a good chance you'll feel like you've gained (blood sugar) superpowers; this is normal. You'll unlock a new way of thinking, of problem-solving, of living life to the fullest. You'll learn all about blood sugar formulas, diabetes shortcuts, and pitfalls to watch out for. You'll learn about the three levels of blood sugar impacts to remove those mysterious and frustrating "blood sugar roller coasters." You'll identify *your* unique strategies and formulas for easier, simpler diabetes management so you can free up some mental space to enjoy more of what life has to offer. You'll even have special access to a few private trainings that I did *for* and *with* my clients to ensure you have everything you need to succeed with your blood sugar.

If you commit to me that you will take action on what I teach, I will not let you fail. I firmly believe that those who read this book will be lifted to an entirely new level of living. These are the same methods that have kept my blood sugar in range more than 90% of the time with an A1C in the high 5s/low 6s for over five years straight while living my life to the fullest as a new dad, husband, triathlete, business owner, world traveler, and foodie. Possibility awaits, and all you have to do right now is read on. I've poured my heart into this book as I do everything in our online educational content. I truly hope this inspires and empowers you to elevate your quality of life and bring more certainty to your blood sugar management.

Note: The countless years of revolutionary information organized in this book were meticulously vetted, consolidated, and streamlined in order to provide the clearest, simplest, and most beneficial path forward for *you* to simplify and master your blood sugar. Do not skip ahead to the chapters that look more fun. Do not read this book out of order or fail to implement the lessons shown. Do *not* put this book away until you have completed every single page and squeezed out every drop of the life-changing, thought-provoking, innovative, and counterintuitive lessons that it has to offer.

This book comes as a direct result of years of research, decades of experimentation, and thousands of lives saved and transformed for the better. I won't lie to you like many others in the diabetes health industry likely already have—this diabetes thing is hard. There's a reason you haven't been able to master your blood sugars—yet. But I promise you that this book will unlock new opportunities and understanding as you read it *if* you implement what you read. Knowledge left unused is knowledge lost and wasted. Prepare yourself for your journey ahead, as life will never be the same after learning how to *think differently* with your diabetes management. I know that's a big promise, so I need the rest of the book to prove it to you. Stick with me and I'll give you everything you need. Let's dive in.

Special Note: *While "blood glucose" is the more scientifically accurate term, you'll see that I refer to it as "blood sugar" throughout this book. As far as my teachings are concerned, I view these two terms as interchangeable (with "blood sugar" being more conversational, hence the decision to primarily use this term).*

CHAPTER 1

MY STORY

On December 23, 2009, near the end of one of the most chaotic months I've ever lived through, I received what was probably the most devastating and depressing news of my entire life. With tears in my eyes, I had taken my childhood dog (and best friend), Shadow, to be put down. A week later, I totaled my car on the freeway in a freak late-night accident where my steering wheel locked up and forced me into the center divide. I failed out of several college classes (both from college "distractions" as well as an overwhelming brain fog that I couldn't yet identify). And then, to wrap up the month of December and welcome me into Christmas, I was diagnosed with type 1 diabetes, and my life was forever changed.

I was in complete shock and disbelief as I didn't know anything about the disease and (embarrassingly) assumed that all diabetics were like the overweight stereotypes we saw on TV. I thought there was no way that a collegiate athlete, someone who has been eating healthy and exercising his entire life, could possibly have diabetes. As it turns out, I'd been fed a mountain of misinformation by the media. There's an autoimmune version that I was unaware of, type 1, that doesn't care how "healthy" you are and will take over your life like a chaotic tornado of frustration and confusion.

From that point forward, I was incredibly angry, confused, and even depressed as I tried to navigate what my life would look like with diabetes. My first response was to shove it down, ignore it, and move on. Even though my first doctor's visit had left me completely void of any hope, I didn't want diabetes to stop me. He told me I would never live a normal life or be able to eat carbohydrates or sugar of any kind again, that I would die within ten years, and that it would be a slow and painful death, including losing limbs, among other diabetic complications. For some reason, my first sad thought was that I wouldn't get to have my favorite chewy chocolate chip granola bar ever again (even considering the supposed *imminent* death looming in my future, I was more worried about my favorite snacks).

Thankfully, growing up in a family that worked in the medical field, we were able to quiet some of the fears wrongly instilled in me (along with identifying that the doctor sent me home without a prescription for fast-acting insulin by mistake—great start by my medical team). We were able to recognize that a life with type 1 diabetes doesn't have to look much different from what was considered a "normal" life. I needed to manage my blood sugar, count my carbs, and take my insulin, but I should be able to live a very full life as long as I managed everything well. I was still angry—and actually depressed—about the diagnosis, but at least I had a new glimmer of hope.

I didn't like being different, though, and to be transparent, I was still "coming out of my shell" at that time in my life (I was incredibly insecure and shy) and just wanted to fit in with the crowd. I didn't need something like a type 1 diabetes diagnosis to make me stand out or make me "special," and I was embarrassed to tell anyone about it. My immediate family knew of my diagnosis, as well as a few close friends, but aside from that, I hid everything from anyone who didn't need to know (including the pancake eating contest that I won without taking any insulin—ask me about this if you end up in one of our programs, it wasn't pretty).

I felt like type 1 diabetes made me weak, and I was embarrassed and insecure. I was a collegiate athlete, right? I felt suddenly humbled and oddly "human" with a disease that brought me to my knees and made me question if I'd ever do anything great in life with such a significant disability. I was reminded that life can be fragile and things can change at a moment's notice. It took me a long time to fully accept my diagnosis as something lifelong, something that I needed to take care of every single day with no breaks or time off. In fact, I didn't initially take care of my blood sugar as well as I should have. I ignored a lot of what was recommended to me. I didn't count my carbs perfectly. I didn't always take my insulin for snacks. Heck, I didn't even test my blood sugar for months on end, and in some cases, there might have been a time when I went even longer without checking. Not too long after being diagnosed with diabetes, I moved across the country from San Diego, California, where I grew up, to New York to try out modeling and see if I could make it in the big city.

While in New York, I got a phone call from my mom one day. She was checking in on me to make sure I was eating my vegetables and getting enough sleep—standard mom stuff. Then, she asked if I had been checking my blood sugar. I paused and responded, "I don't know where my glucometer is." (A glucometer is the device I used to check my blood sugars before wearing the continuous glucose monitor [CGM] that I now have.) She reminded me that she wanted me to take care of myself and be healthy so I'd be around for a longer period of time.

At that time in my life, I lived in what I call a "**stupid fearless**" stage and struggled to prioritize my health. This often meant living my life to the fullest and not letting diabetes hold me back, but doing so in a rather reckless manner. Essentially, this meant not sticking to the recommendations of a life lived well with diabetes, like eating healthy foods, consuming less sugar, taking the proper amount of insulin, and aiming for in-range blood sugar. I was in a very spontaneous phase of my life, and I wanted to get the most out of life *while I still could* (assuming I had only ten years left to live, as my doctor had incorrectly told me).

*****

Learning to Manage My Life With Diabetes

Living life to the fullest (without attentive care for my diabetes) caught up to me over the years. After three or four near-death experiences from emergency low blood sugars, I realized if I didn't take care of this disease, my doctor's initial prediction of an early death filled with diabetes complications might actually come true.

A big part of my journey of attempting to control my diabetes started when my wife and I were first dating. I was living in New York, and she was back in San Diego (long distance relationships are tough), and I came home from work one day after another low blood sugar incident that bounced into a high blood sugar that plummeted into another low (this is what we call the "blood sugar roller coaster"). To be clear, I still wasn't checking my blood sugar levels, but I knew I was high because of the sickness and vomiting. I identified the lows from nearly passing out on the subway as I crammed sugar in my mouth to stop the shaking and sweating. Wreckless.

Already exhausted from the day but more exhausted from managing my blood sugar fluctuations, I stared blankly at the wall after collapsing onto my couch and realized if I didn't figure this thing out, this diabetes thing, there wouldn't be a future with the girl I loved. There would be no family to start with her. I wouldn't be around for my parents or my siblings. That didn't sit right with me. I knew that while I might not pay attention to my blood sugar as much as I should, it was selfish of me to pretend that my life and my experience with diabetes didn't impact the people who love me. I recognized that if I continued the path that I was on—not taking care of myself, not giving it my best—I might never live to see those I love grow old.

I made a commitment at that very moment to take my diabetes seriously, starting with finding my glucometer to see what my blood sugar *actually* was.

As much as I hated that I had diabetes and how unfair it was, I knew I needed to take a step forward and take responsibility for the disease. If this was what life was going to be for me, I had to take action toward creating a successful future instead of remaining complacent. For whatever reason, it set a fire in my heart to start doing the basics, like testing my blood sugar, counting carbs, and taking the proper amount of medication I needed to keep me alive and healthy. I saw that with time and effort, progress and results often followed. Within days, I was feeling better. Weeks later, I felt more energized. Over the following months, my diabetes was less unpredictable, which led to more consistency in my day-to-day living.

As part of my commitment to take care of myself, I went to my doctor and asked for help, but I quickly realized that doctors and endocrinologists are there to help us *survive* with diabetes, but not necessarily to *thrive* with diabetes. Given only a handful of Band-Aid fixes and limited resources from our quick 15-minute appointment, I was faced with the stark realization that I held myself (and my health) to a higher standard than they ever would. "You're doing 'good enough.' No need to make any big changes," they said.

I knew I needed to take this into my own hands, essentially becoming my own doctor, if I expected to live my life in a way I called "**smart fearless.**" I wanted to do the things I love—travel the world and eat the foods I wanted—while maintaining controlled blood sugars that would allow me to live a long, healthy life. I wanted the best of both worlds: happy *and* healthy; who wouldn't want that? And for a while, I thought I knew everything I needed to know about diabetes management because things were indeed "good enough." I was counting my carbs now, I was checking my blood sugars, and I even learned about new devices like a CGM that was dramatically beneficial because I could see my blood sugar updates every five minutes. But even with all these new strategies, devices, knowledge, and research, there was a moment in my life while traveling through Europe as a model (I ended up actually making it into a successful career with TV commercials, music videos with celebrities, billboards, magazine covers and more) where I ran into a terrifying blood sugar scenario that nearly killed me.

*****

My Diabetes Wake-Up Call

While running around Europe (and living there for a brief period of time after getting married to the San Diego love of my life back home, who was "worth figuring out diabetes for"), managing diabetes had its tricky moments. There were times when my insulin was lost with my checked luggage on flights, and I had to run into a local foreign hospital to get new prescriptions on the go. There were times when I didn't have healthy food options or carb counts and had to guess with my insulin dosing.

But a time just outside of Paris, France, stands out above the rest. I had a near-death experience that shook me to my core, and it still haunts me to this day because I don't fully know what went wrong. It was one of those experiences that went *really* wrong, *really fast*. After a day exploring the beautiful city of Paris, I settled into my apartment for the night to get ready for my early morning flight to Italy for another modeling gig. I picked up some food at a local restaurant, ate it, and then noticed something curious about my blood sugar that didn't feel right.

See, for the week prior, I had been experiencing blood sugar that was constantly so high that I was fearful of diabetic ketoacidosis (DKA), a potentially life-threatening complication of diabetes. I had finally gotten my hands on some new insulin (I assumed that was the root cause of my high blood sugar) from a local hospital across the street from the Notre Dame Cathedral (this was before it burned down) and was finally in a healthy blood sugar range again - until this uncertain moment after dinner when my blood sugar started to drop instead of the anticipated rise from the food I'd just consumed. I grabbed some snacks to eat from my backpack, wondering if I'd taken a little too much insulin, but my blood sugar continued to drop. I ate more… and it plummeted.

Something was off, and I could feel it in my blood. I called my wife, who was back in the States after traveling Europe with me for the previous few months. I was confused and nervous about my blood sugar response. My wife heard the urgency in my voice.

It should be noted that, until this point in my life, I was fearless. This was probably the first time my wife had heard an ounce of fear in my voice. Her tone changed immediately, and she went into problem-solver mode. She contacted the host of the Airbnb apartment, who was across the hall, and notified him of my situation. While she was on the phone with him, I searched the house for any kind of food—nothing in the fridge except eggs and cheese. Terror set in as I realized that there were zero shops in the area open this late at night, given that it was such a small town. With no options for additional food, it was time to consider final attempts. I pulled my glucagon out of my backpack, my CGM beeping wildly at me, my wife texting me directions to the nearest hospital, and a confirmation from the Airbnb host that they would take me there if needed.

Sure enough, the Airbnb host opened the door and looked at me with a confused stare. I tried my best to tell him in French that I was ready to go because this was an emergency. He gave me a weird look because I "looked fine" (ugh, this *invisible disease* thing is a killer), but he agreed to take me to the hospital. In the car, I rip open my emergency sugar stash and start cramming some nasty cake icing in my mouth (why can't they make better-tasting, fast-acting sugar?). My CGM reads 60 mg/dL with double arrows down and continuing to drop fast. I'm shaking violently by this point, but I can't tell if it's from the low blood sugar or my new experience with an ongoing panic attack (keep in mind, I've never had a panic attack before in my life). I could still eat sugar, though things were starting to get a little hazy as I wondered how far my blood sugar would drop. I honestly wondered if this was the end for me. We got to the hospital, and my heart sank as I saw the enormous line of people reaching from the front desk to the door; at least 30 people were waiting. I didn't know if help would arrive before it was too late, so I made the bold choice to march straight to the front, nearly collapsing on the way there because my legs felt like jelly at this point.

Getting to the front desk, in a stupor with my legs buckling beneath me, I was met with confused glances from the staff because I was speaking English and they only understood French. In broken French, I made a second attempt. "Je suis diabète. J'ai besoin de sucre," which translates to "I am diabetic and I need sugar." They understood enough, but they couldn't quite grasp the complexity or the seriousness of the situation. I was given a wheelchair because I couldn't stand on my own at this point. I was weak from the blood sugar depletion, couldn't hold myself upright, and the room began to spin. If I passed out, nobody would know what to do to save my life. Panic and hopelessness set in, and I questioned whether I would make it out alive due to this simple communication barrier.

They guided me to the back, where I was given a small glass of water and a single sugar tablet. I told them I needed sugar in an IV, but there was no way I could communicate to them the dire situation I was in; if I didn't receive an enormous amount of sugar in the next 15 minutes, I might die. Instead, they proceeded to take my blood pressure and vitals per protocol before wheeling me to the next room. And once again, my heart sank. I turned white as a ghost as I realized I was not being taken to receive care but to wait in a holding room, forgotten in a room with others who had also been left to wait ages ago. This hospital staff was moving at snails' pace and had no real motivation to speed things up.

I heard the door shut behind me and messaged my wife to give her an update and tell her how much I loved her. She began to panic, realizing that this might be my "goodbye" text, and called me immediately. We walked through potential strategies while she fought back tears, asking what was left in my bag and what else we could do given the circumstances. We refused to give up. Sifting through my backpack, I found a few extra pieces of food that I had not seen before (expired from years earlier, but food nonetheless). I got my glucometer out so I could check my blood sugar numbers. They had continued to drop but had slowed down slightly. Maybe they were stabilizing but still low? I wasn't sure. The world remained blurry, and my mind was slow to function in the absence of substantial glucose as my CGM read 42 mg/dL and was still dropping.

Back in San Diego, my wife had gone to my parents' house by this point because she wanted to let them know the seriousness of the situation and be with others who loved me. My entire family prayed for me and let me know that they were there for me. For the next four hours, I fought my blood sugar levels without being seen once by a doctor, a medical staff member, or even a janitor. The door never opened, the homeless patients locked in the room with me fell asleep long ago, and after hours of exhausting, mortifying, debilitating diabetes difficulties had passed, I had won the fight against severe low blood sugar, scared and alone in a small town of a foreign country. It was one of the most difficult battles of my life.

I checked my blood sugar on my glucometer after watching it skyrocket from under 40 to around 400 in the final hour. The food was finally hitting, and I breathed a sigh of relief, realizing it was probably the first full breath of air I'd taken the whole time that wasn't restricted by anxiety and fear. I texted my wife and let her know I'd walk back to the Airbnb since it wasn't too far. She called again and asked what my plan was.

"Well, I have a flight to Italy in a few hours, so I'm gonna try to get some sleep, and then I'll come home after this next job."

She was livid. "You almost died, and you're gonna stay out there? I *need* you. Come home now."

We went back and forth about finances briefly before ultimately deciding that I should go home to be with her and my family. After all, we still didn't know what happened, and if there was a repeat situation, it might be the actual end of me. (I'd later learn that after an urgent hypoglycemia event, repeat lows are more likely over the following 24 hours). I needed the job in Italy to pay for the bills we had accumulated over the last few months while living in Europe, but she assured me that my life was more important than financial security. "We can figure out the money, but I'm not willing to risk losing you," she said. We spent the last of our savings to get me home on a very expensive last-minute flight back to San Diego, where my entire family met me at the airport, tears welling up in everyone's eyes as we embraced.

After making it out of the hospital in France without ever being seen (furthering my lack of trust in the medical system, both in the U.S. and abroad), I recognized that we are, and forever will be, our own best advocates while living with this invisible illness. We are our own best chance, not only for survival but for a higher quality of life. I recognize now that doctors and medical professionals might have our best interests in mind, but they don't always have the resources, the time, or the ability to help us as much as we are able to help ourselves.

It was at that moment that I knew two things were true. One was that I could not depend solely on my medical team for my care. I needed to take responsibility for this disease and take action in my own way. I couldn't wait any longer. The second was that if I expected to have any quality of life, any peace of mind moving forward, I needed to figure out how to avoid situations like that near-death event in the future. Because if there was any level of uncertainty in my management of diabetes, if I didn't know when the next near-death experience was looming, I would never be able to be fully present. I'd forever wonder if I would make it to another day without another blood sugar surprise. That uncertainty and desperation is what kicked off my passion (more of an obsession, really) to discover every nuanced detail of diabetes and figure out how I could guarantee that I wouldn't be in that kind of situation again.

While on that emergency flight home—on which I spent our savings (remember, she insisted that I take the flight)—there was a moment that sparked a new passion project for me. Although, as I previously mentioned, it can be better marked by obsession and desperation as I battled for mental peace and certainty. Through this process, I became fascinated with blood sugar science. I needed to understand why blood sugar did what it did and, more importantly, *how to make it do what I wanted it to do* so I could avoid dangerous situations while still living my life to the fullest. So, for the next two years, I dedicated myself, my resources, my money, my time, and 100% of my energy toward identifying what would eventually become known as the

"**80/20 Blood Sugar Formula.**" It was a way to not only understand what blood sugar does but to learn how to predict stable blood sugars, how to manipulate blood sugars that aren't cooperating as we'd like them to, and how to keep blood sugars so stable that we're able to finally live our lives again. A way to live happy *and* healthy.

Note: The 80/20 Blood Sugar Formula is what we now set up (fully customized to each individual) with my private coaching clients living with type 1 diabetes, and it allows us to act with confidence and certainty with our blood sugar plan in order to keep blood sugar "in check" while we live our life on our terms. What makes the 80/20 Blood Sugar Formula unique from the other formulas that we'll walk through together in this book is that it allows us to set up quick exchanges with *actual* calculations for more precise management of blood sugar.

Using this formula, I can tell you with near-certainty where blood sugars will end up after a meal, what will happen to them during or after exercise, and even how many carbs I need in order to "bump" my blood sugar up 17 points (or however many points I need to elevate them in that moment). It turns the "guessing game" of diabetes into a simple sequence that builds on top of what I'll teach you in this book. It makes diabetes make sense. Precise prediction = control that I could depend on. However, as I'm sure you already know, diabetes looks *very* different for all of us, so that level of precision control does need to be personalized (which is what I specialize in with my clients). That process, gaining more certainty with blood sugar management, was also a bit therapeutic for me as I fought my way through some of the hardest mental struggles of my life—anxiety, depression, suicidal ideation, panic attacks bordering on agoraphobia (the fear of going outside of "safe" places like my home), and a fear of being alone—coming from a man who was previously labeled as fearless by all who knew him.

After my near-death experience just outside of Paris, my diabetes management strategies had shifted from "doing fine and getting by" to operating and making decisions out of absolute terror and fear. I was so scared of low blood sugar and large doses of insulin that I ran my blood sugar high all the time. My endocrinologist saw that my blood sugar was pretty consistently sitting in the 200s and 300s and sometimes even higher and made a point to pull me aside and talk to me about it. I asked her if it was really that big of a deal to keep my blood sugar high, even if only for a few weeks while I got my bearings and regained comfort with dosing "normal" amounts of insulin again. She looked disgusted and said, "Absolutely not. You're killing yourself! This will have an impact on your health, and you need to take this seriously." I needed a reset, and I needed help.

*****

Using Restrictions to Manage My Diabetes

After the reality check with my endo, I did bring my average blood sugar down, but the strategies I used to get it there were not the best. In fact, initially, my entire strategy was to live in complete restriction. I restricted fun, I restricted activity, I restricted travel, and above all else, I restricted food. I fell into a hyper-restrictive diet protocol, which led me to try low-carb—bordering on keto but not quite—because I was scared to take large amounts of insulin for meals in fear that it might push me into another low blood sugar episode.

After I tried low-carb and near-keto diets, I found a new popular diet that recommended low-fat, whole-food plant-based as the way to go. I experimented with that, and it did lead to improved insulin sensitivity, but it also caused massive blood sugar fluctuations that scared me even more. I was taking 70% less insulin (*which, I mean, wow, right?*), but the insulin that I did take seemed to be a bit like taking a ride on a roller coaster because of how fast it worked. After a few months of giving it my best, I once again found myself in an emergency blood sugar situation while I was filming a music video in the Hollywood Hills area for a very well-known movie series. I ended up being "that guy" on set who had an ambulance called for him in the middle of the music video shoot. How embarrassing it was to show up as one of the lead characters in a music video and to then be walked off the set by firefighters and paramedics with what seemed like "nothing" going on because nobody could "see" anything wrong with me. They couldn't see my blood sugar plummeting or the terror in my eyes (thanks to PTSD, another invisible condition).

As fear held a tight grip on me day to day—especially with a repeat event fresh in my memory—I shrunk into fear more and more, enjoying less of life, being less of who I was, and having less will to live. I was so scared to "upset" my diabetes that I found myself restricting my quality of life. I was afraid to go to restaurants that didn't have "diabetic-friendly" food. Once more, just like many years earlier in New York, I realized that I wasn't controlling my diabetes; diabetes was controlling me. All the effort I was putting in was yielding an A+ on my diabetes report card with my A1C and time in range looking stellar, but I was miserable and exhausted. And while my blood sugar looked decent and I was getting high-fives from my medical team, I had essentially built for myself a "diabetes prison." I did what was necessary to keep my blood sugar from going low or going high, but it came at the sacrifice of living a fulfilling life. It felt like I was making plans, decisions, and excuses for my diabetes. In other words, I was living *for* my diabetes, not with it. For everything that I wanted to do, I had to check on my numbers first to see if my blood sugar would "let" me participate.

Looking back, I can tell you that my wife and my family suffered as a result as well. I was a walking nervous wreck, staring at my CGM every four and a half minutes, waiting for the clock to hit five minutes so I could get my updated blood sugar and feel a sense of relief that my number was "safe," at least until the next update in four and a half minutes. My family couldn't rely on me for anything, and while I didn't know it at the time, I was a burden. I was fragile. I was a different person from the man they once knew. Months later, I recognized this and knew I couldn't live my life like this long term. My mental fragility, my desperation for blood sugar control, and my hyper-restrictive strategies were not a long-term play. It wasn't realistic, and I saw that it was hurting those I loved as well as myself.

So, I set out to discover a new method for blood sugar mastery because the current traditional methods—even the cutting-edge methods of the day with new dietary protocols—were not working for me. I felt like I had a different version of diabetes that was more difficult and in need of more specialized attention, and I wanted to hold myself to a higher standard than "just surviving" with diabetes.

*****

Diabetes and My Mental Health

I was someone who had traveled to thirty-six countries, even journeying through Europe with nothing more than a small backpack and my wits to guide me. But for the first time in my life, I was now mentally broken and had fallen much further than I had ever thought possible. I had never experienced anxiety or panic attacks before, but now they were a daily occurrence, and I was a completely different person—and not in a good way—which made sense with the PTSD diagnosis I had gotten from my medical team after returning home. I had become someone who was nervous about even going outside. For the first time ever, diabetes had limited my ability to live my life as I wanted to, and I worried it would be the thing to take me out after all those years of traveling, playing sports, and living my best life. I had hit rock bottom. No, it was deeper than rock bottom; I felt like I had been buried *underneath* the rocks at rock bottom and was being suffocated by the sheer pressure of life. I realized that I now had a choice to make after spending a few weeks at home after the incident: either settle into my new "home" beneath rock bottom or choose to push through and claw my way out of the hellish hole my mind had put me into.

When I was in my **"stupid fearless"** stage, I put on a strong face, but I was filled with anger, depression, and anxiety, and I was uncertain of my future. The doctors I went to for help offered temporary fixes but no permanent solutions. It took five years of trying to force diabetes to work with their cookie-cutter approach for me to realize that I had to take care of it myself, create my own rules, and be a **"renegade warrior,"** so to speak. Only after that did I begin to understand the complexity of diabetes and the reasons why it was so difficult to control. After my near-death experience in Paris, I came back to the States with a new challenge, which was not to remove diabetes from my life but to learn how to live in harmony with it by keeping my blood sugar controlled, finally allowing me to live my best healthy life without diabetes getting in the way or holding me back.

So, I researched. I experimented on my blood sugar daily. I connected with medical teams in experimental branches far and wide, looking for a cure or a revolutionary treatment option. I searched online medical databases. I became obsessed (unhealthily, I'll admit) with blood sugar management. I became so hyper-focused on blood sugar variables and creating my own methods for mastering this beast of a disease that my wife and family had to request that I *not* talk about diabetes at the dinner table and at family get-togethers. I was in the zone and taking note of *every* detail I encountered. I felt like a mad scientist and even quit my job so that I could devote 100% of my time and energy to this.

I wasn't right in the head, but I *needed* certainty in my blood sugar again. My wife supported me as long as I was making progress through my mental health struggles. She encouraged me to see a therapist, which I did. However, the way I saw it, if I could come up with something that allowed me to predict where blood sugar was *going to go* and *if* I could master diabetes as a whole, I'd finally have my life back. Peace of mind, schedule flexibility, and the freedom to eat, do, and experience whatever I wanted would directly result from my blood sugar being so well controlled. At least, that was the goal.

Over the course of two years of daily experimentation, research, trial and error, and so much more, I was able to discover patterns and answers and finally create an organization of blood sugar management methods and formulas that allowed me to keep blood sugar exactly where I wanted it, give me back my mental peace, and to give me hope for a future where I'd be able to have spontaneity, adventure, and fun once again.

As I shifted into living my life as what I consider "**smart fearless**," diabetes looked very different. I had learned over many years that if I ignored my diabetes, it would remind me it was still there with lows and highs and out-of-control experiences, almost as if it were demanding my attention. But if I kept it controlled and in line, I was free to live my life without distraction or interruption. I realized that if I wanted to live my best life, I couldn't ignore my diabetes. I had to pay attention to it and respect its dangerous potential to protect myself from having any more near-death experiences.

66 ———————————————

Living with diabetes is like running a race with no finish line. There will not be an end, and so we must endure.

——————————————— **99**

This book is a collection of the lessons learned through those grueling two years and the shortcuts to success and stable blood sugar that I'm now able to offer you as a result of making it out on the other side of blood sugar mastery. I've done my best to consolidate and simplify, and I'm thrilled to have you here reading this book. Especially because in the next chapter, we will be breaking down some commonly held false beliefs you might have heard from your medical team and diving right into what you can do to fix them. In fact, before we go any further, I'll share that it's not just about the A1C, as our medical teams often insist. As it turns out, that's only the *first step* of four (as you'll see in the image below) that we take our private clients through. In this book, I'll be walking with you step by step as we explore these revolutionary new methods that simplify diabetes management on a more personalized level, recognizing you as an individual with diabetes, not just as another "diabetic patient."

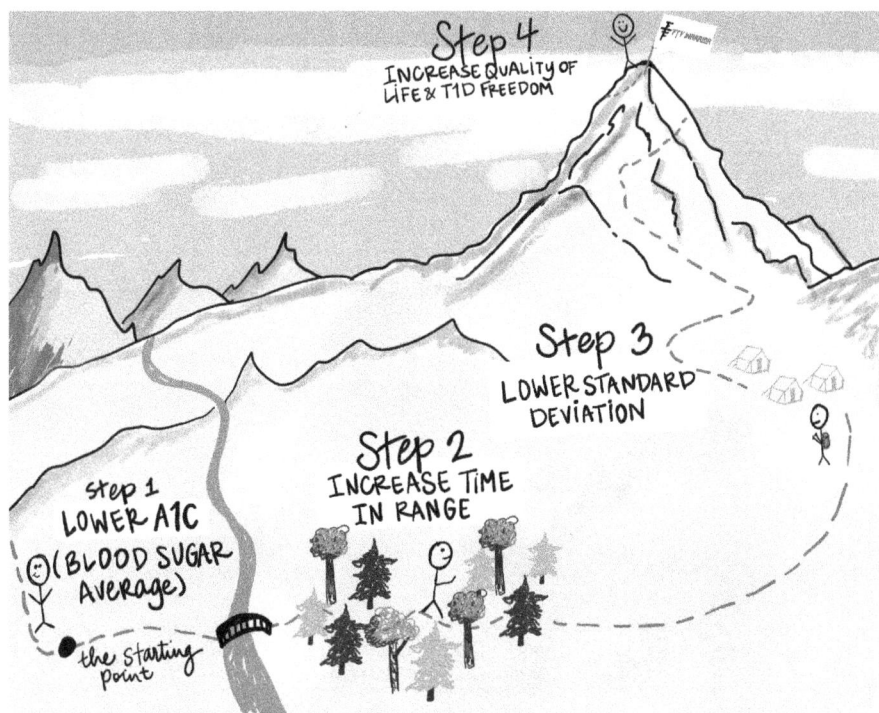

It's only when we *think differently* that we experience all that we were meant to in life. And you were meant for so much more (see Step #4 in the image above).

Notes:

_____

_____

_____

_____

_____

_____

_____

_____

_____

_____

_____

_____

_____

_____

_____

_____

_____

_____

CHAPTER 2

YOU'VE BEEN LIED TO

Back when I was finally ready to address my diabetes and take it seriously, I spent some time getting to know my medical team. My endocrinologist was the first stop as I had lots of questions about why I was seeing my blood sugar creep up throughout the day, in between meals, and overnight. I noticed my average blood sugar was higher than I would like it to be, and I wondered if it was impacting my A1C. My endo had a pretty straightforward approach and agreed that my high blood sugar between meals needed to be dealt with. Adding more long-acting insulin was the suggestion, and unfortunately, this is something common in a lot of T1D clients I take on these days. That's not to say that it's automatically wrong to make that adjustment, but you'll soon see why this is a common mistake made in the medical world (and how to fix it).

Oftentimes, we see this "if-then" relationship for decision-making without any context being asked (or given) before making adjustments to insulin in many endo and primary care offices. Ultimately, my endocrinologist saw that I had high blood sugars that were seemingly unrelated to my meals because of how "far away" it was from my mealtime dose, concluded that I needed more long-acting insulin as a result, and sent me on my way without looking any deeper.

The issue that I would later learn is that simply adding more insulin does not solve all high blood sugar problems, nor is it even the first stop in many cases. What ended up happening is that we added too much long-acting insulin (I was on Lantus at the time, though I wear an insulin pump now), and I found myself going low every single night from that moment forward. I'd wake up in a pool of sweat, shaking and confused, crawl to the fridge to drink a juice box, and drag myself back into bed. This caused me to develop a fear of the unknown, of what might happen while I was asleep—sometimes, I even questioned if I'd wake up in the morning. My daytime blood sugar looked fine, so the endocrinologist was able to fix the problem on a surface level, but my quality of life was suffering, and I was "feeding the insulin" (when taking too much insulin, we're forced to constantly snack in an effort to avoid oncoming lows). Her recommendation to fix the nighttime time lows? "Just have a snack before bed every night." Great, another quick fix. What's worse is that I looked good "on paper" because my A1C was lower, but it was only an average and didn't take into account the day-to-day struggles and frustration with little to no sleep.

What many endocrinologists and doctors give us are often just surface-level Band-Aid fixes to get us "back on our feet" and out of their offices. They've taught us incorrectly how to manage our diabetes by treating only the symptoms. If we're being honest, this approach likely stems from the medical education system teaching them incorrectly in the first place. Our medical teams are, in many cases, misinformed by *their* educators or just using old and outdated methods and strategies, which leads to them teaching that same outdated information to us (not knowing that it is outdated). Then there is the pressure put on practitioners to produce results—the "more patients = more money" mode of operation—that can cause providers to become negligent. When the medical staff charged with our care aren't equipped to (or able to) address our frustrations or concerns, it can leave us feeling hopeless and alone. As I've discovered, we have to learn to advocate and fend for ourselves, and we must take responsibility for our diabetes management and subsequent outcomes—both good *and* bad.

Oftentimes, the recommendations coming from our endocrinologists, dietitians, doctors, and other medical professionals are those from decades past, where restrictive diets, lifestyles, and schedules were the "go-to" diabetes advice. The recommendation was to always eat the same thing, take the same insulin at the same time of day, and limit your spontaneity and fun (blah blah blah), and hypothetically, you'd be just fine. For the record, this was actually a good idea… once upon a time. Back before we had CGMs to give us constant updates on our numbers every five minutes, insulin pumps for personalized precision dosing, or "smart" insulin pens, it was nearly impossible to have stable blood sugar without a consistent and restricted lifestyle.

Let's revisit my endo's quick-fix error before moving on. As an example of addressing the root cause (instead of slapping on a Band-Aid fix), let's compare it to an old car I used to have—my first car, actually. It was a 1986 Honda Accord with a manual gearbox (it was a stick shift) that my grandpa gave to me. It had something like 300,000 miles on it (he took *really* good care of it), and there were certain "quirks" that came with that car. Here's a fun one: the power steering fluid would just "disappear" every few weeks, and I'd have to carry around spare power steering fluid in the trunk so I could refill it periodically. No big deal… unless I forgot to refill it, which could be life-threatening since I'd no longer have the ability to safely steer my car. But had I gone a little deeper and figured out what was actually going on instead of just fixing the "symptoms," I might have been able to help the car live even longer, I wouldn't have been in constant danger of forgetting something critical, *and* I would have saved a ton of money over the years not having to buy power steering fluid every few weeks.

If we only treat the symptoms (like my endo and the high blood sugars or my car with the leaky steering fluid), we rarely get to actually move on from that problem; it requires we give it continued "maintenance" and attention. This can lead to us feeling like we're constantly "babysitting" our blood sugar to make sure that it doesn't do anything crazy or unpredictable. The answer here for many of us who find ourselves in this situation is to micromanage our diabetes, which does "work," but it can get exhausting and lead to burnout and a poor quality of life in the long run.

*****

Treating Symptoms is Only the Beginning

The other issue with the blood sugar strategies that just fix the symptoms is that life for most of us is not consistent enough for that to work. We have things that come up, we have new experiences, and we get pulled in different directions by work, family, or spontaneity. For example, I recently became a parent (a few years ago), and things look a little different now when I go to eat a meal (or do anything for that matter). In addition to running a business, traveling the world, and being an athlete, things like this can take us out of a "diabetes routine" and force us into a more dynamic approach where a blood sugar formula might make more sense to rely on (more on that soon). The issue is that our doctors and endocrinologists don't teach us anything about a dynamic approach. They teach us more in the realm of *if-then* statements. *If* blood sugar is high, *then* take insulin. *If* blood sugar is low, *then* eat sugar. But diabetes is so much more than "if this happens, then do that." What if I have insulin on board? What if there's a dessert that I want to eat after I've finished my meal? What if my blood sugars never stay steady and in range? What if, what if, what if?

Often, this leads us to either restrict our choices (because it doesn't fit in with the *if-then* method we've been taught) or dive headfirst into new territory, like trying to tackle dosing insulin for pizza and hoping for the best. These gaps in knowledge can lead to dangerous pitfalls when guessing, especially when trying to live a semi-normal life, deciding which strategies to use for insulin dosing, or how to manage blood sugar that isn't cooperating when the "plan" doesn't work as intended. Consider the multiple trips to the hospital in my own past as lessons learned from my own trial and error - I'd like to help you avoid those dangers as much as possible if you can learn from my mistakes over the last decade as you read this book.

Ultimately, the gaps that exist in your diabetes management are not your fault but rather the fault of a system that has failed us. A system that found something that worked "good enough" for the masses decades ago and continues to teach it now without much improvement. It's the same system that refuses to update its methods, research, or options for what life can look like *today* with diabetes. What you currently know about diabetes is incomplete at a foundational level because your medical team is likely either using outdated information or doesn't have enough time to actually personalize an action plan with you. But what can you do about it? What doctors have taught us in the past does work to a certain extent and can manage blood sugar, but only through restriction and consistency—so let's discuss how to break free from the mold of complacency and mediocrity.

What we've learned over the years is that it's not just about insulin-to-carb ratios, but proteins and fats and fibers, the glycemic index, and an entire list of other blood sugar variables that must be considered. If we're being honest, that knowledge gap is likely the reason you're experiencing wacky levels that your doctor can't identify. My endocrinologist decided to increase my long-acting insulin to fix the high blood sugars, though we can now identify it as a delayed spike from high-protein and high-fat meals that I was eating. It's time we identify and fix the source, not just the symptoms. [*Think Differently*]

When my doctor made the change in my insulin to fix the high blood sugars, thinking it was from a low long-acting dose, she put me at risk for overnight lows that resulted in me chasing my blood sugar every single night. Why did that happen, though? As I've discovered from my research many years later (and as I mentioned above), my daily high blood sugar was the result of a high-fat and high-protein diet. Since I only needed additional fast-acting insulin to fix the highs during the day (when I ate food), the increase in long-acting insulin worked as long as I was eating but created new problems (lows) when I skipped meals or slept overnight.

This is because long-acting insulin (also called "basal" insulin for insulin pump users) is meant to cover 24 hours as a baseline, whereas my needs in this specific example only called for localized (fast-acting) additional insulin to cover my post-meal highs. I could have taken a second dose of fast-acting insulin at a specified time after meals to counteract this and found my solution (more on that later) without increasing my risk for overnight lows. Because no two diabetics are the same, there is no cookie-cutter plan for diabetes management. This, of course, makes it tricky and requires that we play an active role in managing our blood sugar. If we can identify the root cause of what's going wrong (like the fats and proteins in this example), we can then find a solution that matches our situation without making things worse. This is where critical thinking comes into play.

The bad news is that I need you to forget 90% of what you've been led to believe about type 1 diabetes and replace it with the practical knowledge from this book, along with the updated and new additional resources provided. The good news is that I'm here to guide you through the revolutionary new strategies, blood sugar formulas, counterintuitive methods, and more. A phrase that has served me well over the years when researching new strategies and implementing new plans is that "nothing changes if nothing changes." In other words, if we expect a new outcome (like more controlled blood sugars), we're probably going to have to try some new strategies because, clearly, what we've been doing so far isn't working. That being said, I want to acknowledge that growth is uncomfortable. We have been previously taught that high blood sugar means more insulin is needed, and low blood sugar means more sugar is needed—as if those were our only options. The truth is that there are far more variables that push and pull blood sugars up and down, and when we learn to identify them and *use them strategically*, we're able to not only control blood sugars more regularly but do so with predictability and consistency *while living our best lives.*

Over many years of coaching and helping thousands of other type 1 diabetics like us, my team and I have come across more than 50 variables that impact blood sugar, both up and down. We've also discovered equations that allow us to balance our blood sugar throughout our lives without getting lost in complexity or conflicting information. The difficulty is in the complexity of discovering these equations on your own. And when I talk about "diabetes math" (like formulas and equations) I know it can seem overwhelming—like you're getting tossed back into a math class and that you might fall behind if you don't understand the new concepts. I've got good news, though: just like you wouldn't be thrown into an advanced calculus class if you don't yet understand pre-algebra, I won't introduce anything you're not ready for as you read.

Consider this book an introduction to the foundations of this simple methodology we call "diabetes math." If you can do simple addition and subtraction, I promise that you'll be able to use the strategies outlined in this book without getting lost. I even hired a professional illustrator to add drawings throughout this book for the visual learners who like to see the examples (or if you have ADHD like me and need something to retain your attention).

*****

Surviving Versus Thriving With Diabetes

Let's jump back to our medical teams. Doctors help us *survive* with diabetes—that part is clear, and they're quite good at it. But if we ever expect to *thrive* with diabetes, that's on us.

Unfortunately, the medical system is set up for efficiency (seeing as many patients as possible), not effectiveness (getting you to your *best* life with diabetes). It's just not going to happen. They're often using outdated methods that require us to be ridiculously consistent and static in our approach to diabetes. The strategies they teach ask for yes or no answers (like "Are blood sugars high? Then take more insulin") when what we need is more of an "it depends" approach (you'll learn this later in the book, but context *really* matters with blood sugar decisions and is likely a big part of the reason your blood sugars aren't behaving as well as you'd like). We have to have context when making all of our diabetes management decisions because it truly does depend on things like time of day, how much insulin is on board from a recent bolus, food digestion speed, recent exercise, and even the temperature and humidity outside (yes, I'm serious).

Diabetes management is not black and white. There is a very wide "gray zone" that we have to consider when making decisions for our diabetes management, meaning that there are only a handful of absolute truths we can say definitively impact all diabetics the same. Let's pull an example from something our medical teams believe to be an absolute truth—the rule of 15 for treating low blood sugars. They'll share that for low blood sugar (below 70 mg/dL), they recommend 15 grams of fast-acting carbohydrates, wait 15 minutes, and recheck to see where your blood sugar is after eating. If you're still below 70, eat 15 more grams, wait 15 minutes, and recheck. This is incorrect as a blanket statement. Adding *context*—like knowing how much insulin we have on board, if there was recent activity, or if I just finished a meal—allows me to understand if I need a full 15 grams of sugar to fix this, maybe just 5 grams, or maybe more than 30. The solution changes depending on the *context* of each situation we find ourselves in.

The issue with black-and-white diabetes rules and treating every situation the same is that we often miss the mark and still experience highs and lows more frequently than necessary. In this example, If I were 69 mg/dL and *stable* with zero insulin on board and hanging out on the couch, I'd likely only need a small bite of something (or some people might not choose to do anything about it if they feel fine). Alternatively, if I were at 69 mg/dL and dropping rapidly (like double arrows down on my CGM) with five units of insulin on board and in the middle of a workout, I might consider a much more aggressive response with 30 grams of carbs (or more). Context is KEY.

We can't trust these outdated, static methods of diabetes management because diabetes itself is not static (nor is life, right?). Our blood sugars are going to respond differently on a day-to-day basis. Therefore, our strategies need to change daily as well. We must be able to adapt to new information and make decisions in a dynamic sense. If, for example, I typically eat very healthy, but on the weekend, I go to a holiday party and stuff myself with junk food, my blood sugar is likely to respond very differently, and what works during the week might not work during the weekend as a result. If I'm generally very inactive during the week while sitting behind a desk, but I'm a "weekend warrior," and I'm outside exercising and exploring… guess who's going to be low all weekend from the added activity if I don't change my strategies to match the situation? Knowing what to expect and matching them with different strategies allows me to enjoy more flexibility in life, whether it's a lazy weekend getaway or competing in my next Ironman race. Knowledge of what's new can offer so much more than just survival. It's time to learn new methods that will equip you to actually live your life to the fullest and thrive with diabetes!

The reality (if you haven't caught on just yet) is that adaptation is the name of the game when it comes to diabetes management. If you can adapt to whatever blood sugar variables are thrown your way, you will experience more stability and consistency with your blood sugar *while living life on your terms*. It's either that or following all of the doctor's recommendations of restriction and consistency with robotic commitment, which for most of us is not realistic long term (or enjoyable).

Why trust me, though? We'll skip over the "certified master fitness trainer and nutritionist" piece for now, and we don't even need to explore the keynote speaker, presenter, and even ambassador roles I've enjoyed over the years with the Juvenile Diabetes Research Foundation (JDRF, now called "Breakthrough T1D"), the American Diabetes Association (ADA), Connected in Motion, Beyond Type 1, Tandem Diabetes, Dexcom, and more. Instead, I want to share a bit about the many years I've researched and studied blood sugar variables and how I've come to realize the absolute complexity of this disease while discovering how to finally fix them.

*****

Searching for Solutions

After returning home from what we now refer to as the "Paris incident" (Chapter 1), I essentially turned into a mad scientist obsessed with finding (or creating) a solution to these erratic and unpredictable blood sugar episodes I'd experienced so often as a result of diabetes being so complicated and widely misunderstood. It might sound scary at first thought to hear that it's more complex than you may have previously thought (because you're reading this book to learn about the ins and outs of diabetes, no doubt). But I can promise you that the more we understand how blood sugars work, the more we are able to fill our diabetes toolbox with different options to handle each unique situation.

That phase of my life was critical because it gave me insight into my own diabetes, but over the years of coaching and helping thousands of other insulin-dependent diabetics in our coaching programs, I've had the opportunity to see patterns unfold at scale and show me how the complexities of diabetes can be simplified for just about anyone in any situation. For example, I've already hinted that there are more options to manipulate blood sugars than just insulin and sugar. More options mean more flexibility, which allows for a more adaptive method as we live *with* diabetes, not *for* diabetes. It's almost like trying to build a house with nothing but a hammer and nails. Can you get the job done? Sure, but the best you'll end up with is a shack to keep you protected from the rain, and best of luck to you if the job calls for a specialized tool that you don't have on hand.

However, if you've got a truck full of options—a screwdriver, sander, reciprocating and circular saws, measurement and leveling tools, an actual blueprint to follow, and a template to reference from someone else's successful house build—you're able to build something truly magnificent while overcoming any obstacles along the way with confidence and certainty. When we understand this *context* of the blood sugar movement (and know which diabetes "tool" to use and when), we're able to manipulate the outcomes with our **"diabetes toolbelt"** using strategies (and formulas) we have at the ready in order to build that dream life you've always wanted.

Over the years, I discovered that there are patterns behind our blood sugar, that there are meanings behind the lows *and the highs*, and, most importantly, that every single blood sugar we encounter happens for a reason. There is no such thing as a blood sugar reading without meaning. When we understand that everything that happens to our blood sugar is a series of breadcrumbs (like clues) for us to follow, we can begin to learn from the highs and lows, identify patterns, map out our unique experiences, and eventually learn to predict stable blood sugar using blood sugar formulas. Now, when I say "diabetes math" and blood sugar formulas and equations, it might sound scary because it's an unfamiliar topic, but as I promised earlier, if you're able to handle 1+1=2 kinda math, this method will work for you.

I can say this with confidence because, in my experience with diabetes, I've been let down by my medical team on multiple occasions. I've lived the terror of being scared to go to sleep and wondering if I'd wake up in the morning. I've been forced to stay up into the early morning hours because of blood sugar alerts and alarms, even when all I wanted was to sleep. Just like you, I've yelled at my diabetes and said things I didn't mean to loved ones out of "blood sugar frustration." I've had stubborn high blood sugars that seemed to be so stuck that I questioned if my insulin was bad, and I've battled the lows that seemed unending when I didn't know if I'd make it out alive. I've sat and pondered, *Why me? Why can't it just make sense?* I've been on the "blood sugar roller coaster" with multiple highs and lows on the same day, bouncing back and forth against my will like a kid in a trampoline park getting "super-bounced" by the big kid bullies.

We've been told a lie by our medical teams that diabetes should be "easy," and if it's not, well, "that's just how it is." Our concerns with diabetes complications are either silenced and ignored because we're doing "good enough" or weaponized in an effort to make us more "compliant." We leave the semi-annual endo appointment with a general goal to "improve" but little to no strategy for actual actions that we can take to better our health. We finally decide to take care of ourselves and put some effort in, only to be told, "You're doing 'good enough,'" or "Stop trying so hard," or "That's as good as it gets" as our dreams of living a normal life are quieted. Even if we manage to snag a few "tricks" to try out, it still feels like we're living in a prison of restrictions and rules that hold us back from achieving true health and happiness. If any of this resonates with you, then you are in the right place, and by the end of this book, you will have earned your title of "renegade warrior" alongside the rest of us. Welcome to the rebellion. I'm stoked to have you here on this journey with us.

That being said, what's the actual difference between what you might learn from your doctor's office and from this book that you picked off the shelf? In Chapters 3 and 5, I'll break down the "behind-the-scenes" secrets of your medical team's appointment strategies so that you can use them for yourself. And while most medical teams have books and binders filled with cookie-cutter methods that worked "good enough" in the past, this book was written by someone in the trenches who lives with type 1 diabetes while researching, experimenting, and battling through the day-to-day complexities of living with this disease. I've spent the better part of a decade learning, failing, iterating, innovating, and perfecting the strategies that I've painstakingly organized and consolidated into this book in simplified form. Once you read about and implement these strategies that have already helped thousands of others to succeed, I promise you that life (and life with diabetes) will never be the same.

Here are some free bonuses for buying my book:

- 5-Day Blood Sugar Formula Challenge 2.0
- "Decade in a Document" - Coach Matt's Top Tips
- Renegade Warrior's Manifesto // Renegade Warrior's Newsletter

SCAN THE QR CODE

Notes:

_____

_____

_____

_____

_____

_____

_____

_____

_____

_____

_____

_____

_____

_____

_____

_____

_____

_____

CHAPTER 3

WHAT GETS MEASURED GETS MANAGED

When I first began my journey toward becoming a certified master fitness trainer and nutritionist, my teacher had us begin with an experimental documentation process to identify what our current diet looked like (so that we'd be familiar with analyzing and creating meal plans as we took on clients in the future). The first time I started tracking my food and everything that went into my mouth, I discovered something that continues to shock me to this day. See, when I was first getting into the world of fitness and nutrition, I was completely ignorant of everything it entailed, and one of the main reasons I chose to pursue this path was to gain a deeper understanding of things that impacted my blood sugar and how I might better manage it for my overall health. I knew that I eventually wanted to help people with their health in some capacity, though I had no idea how deep this journey would take me. However, while studying nutrition and logging my food, even for just a couple of days, I found out that I consumed enough fat in a single meal (breakfast) to last an average human multiple days.

You see, my breakfast many years ago used to consist of two egg burritos and coffee. To make those two egg burritos, I would go through a dozen eggs, two handfuls of cheese, and a whole avocado, plus my coffee had melted butter in it (this was when bulletproof coffee was gaining popularity). So, when you take all of that and break it down, it's pretty easy to see how I was consuming over 115 grams of fat (that's over 1,000 calories from the fat in my breakfast *alone*, not even considering the carbs and proteins). The most shocking part about this is that I had been consuming that breakfast for around six months, and it never occurred to me that I might be eating too much fat. This isn't to say that you can't eat that much fat; it was just a shocking realization that showed me that my ignorance and my behavior (when allowed to go unchecked) might lead me toward undesired outcomes like weight gain or insulin resistance.

In fact, the topic that I want to discuss in this chapter, "What gets measured gets managed," can be seen in just about any area of life. We'll take weight loss as an example since our second assignment in my certification training was to track calories and weight fluctuation throughout the week. If you have a general goal of weight loss yet refuse to weigh yourself, look in a mirror, or take body fat percentage measurements, it will often limit the progress that's made because you can't see what works and what doesn't. It's incredibly difficult to identify what's working and what's not when there is no measurement or tracking in place, especially when you're considering the numerical values behind progress (like pounds lost or blood sugars that are in range). If I don't track it, how will I know if I'm losing (or *gaining)* fat?

It's the same with blood sugar management; you'll never know if your blood sugar is getting worse or better if you don't track the outcomes. If you're not watching things like time in range, your A1C, standard deviation, or fasting blood glucose, you'll never know if you're even on the right track. This is the pitfall that I fell into for *years* when I was first diagnosed. I was living in an "ignorance is bliss" mindset, not realizing how bad things were actually getting. It's critical for us to understand why our blood sugar is getting better or worse over time so that we can make adjustments to the things that are hurting our progress and duplicate the things that are working well. It's nearly impossible to identify these trends, however, if we're not tracking our inputs and data along the way. So, when I consider a fasting glucose of 250 mg/dL, I want to know *why* that blood sugar is so high and not just blindly take more insulin as was previously recommended to me by my medical team (again, treating the symptom instead of getting curious about the root cause of the problem).

Instead of just piling on extra medication, I might consider the fact that I used to wake up in the middle of the night and have a snack before going back to bed and then not take insulin for that snack. That might be why my fasting blood sugars are so high. Or maybe it's the "dawn phenomenon" coming to wreak havoc on my blood sugar at the start of each day. Maybe it's the poor quality of sleep. Maybe it's because I skipped my workouts for three days in a row, and it's starting to catch up with me. But if I'm not tracking my fasting blood glucose (and other variables) to begin with, I won't know if that's my norm or if it's a new variable I need to consider. One of the most powerful things that I can teach you in this chapter is to collect data and document it in order to identify trends and patterns (especially because we are all a little different from each other).

When I started to track my fat consumption, I recognized that the amount of fat I was consuming wasn't serving me well in blood sugar management. Unbeknownst to me at the time, it was also destroying my fitness goals. I had always wanted to hit 200 pounds of muscle (honestly, I wanted it because I thought the number 200 sounded cool because I like even numbers), but I had a hard time putting on muscle because my personalized macronutrient profile (PMP) was completely incorrect in order to do what I wanted it to do. I had no idea because I wasn't tracking—or even aware of—my food.

As I began to track and monitor my consumption of different foods and adjust based on the data I collected, my physique began to change. As I began to track my weight on the scale, do caliper tests, and measure body fat percentage, I noticed near-immediate progress and benefits with my lifestyle changes. In the end, tracking macronutrients and blood sugar, along with hydration, sleep hours, and many other variables, allowed me to see *more* progress than I would have seen without it. *I know...* it sounds tedious and boring. But if you can commit to tracking even just a few things while you read this book, I promise you'll make faster and longer-lasting progress toward your goals. For most people like you and me who live with diabetes, that might look like a lower fasting blood sugar level, lower A1C, increased time in range, and even a lower standard deviation (more stable blood sugars).

Let's look at another example. Imagine a large cruise ship heading straight out into the ocean for a grand adventure. While all of the fancy equipment and dashboards have brought us a long way from needing to navigate the open seas by using the stars at night, there's still a *constant* need for observing new information and adjusting the course. Let's say that the ship is headed from my nearest home port of Long Beach, CA to travel toward Tokyo, Japan. Do you think that they're just going to point the ship in the right general direction and hope it lands somewhere around Tokyo? Absolutely not! But this is so often how I see people pursuing their goals in life. "I need to lower my A1C, so I guess I'll just take more insulin." I hear this from both type 1 diabetics *and* their medical teams. Sure, more insulin might be part of the puzzle, but how much more? When? Why? What if you take too much and go low?

So, a cruise ship sailing all over the world isn't going to rely solely on the initial strategy of being pointed in the right direction but also on multiple points of data at frequent intervals throughout the entire voyage. Let's say location, nautical speed, water currents, wind patterns, and so forth are checked once per day. That means that once per day, they have the chance to interpret the data (their inputs) and adjust their course little by little to stay on track toward their destination (their outputs). Compare that to the ship that only checks once per week. They'd likely be completely off course by the time they checked the maps and have to redirect completely, probably losing *days* backtracking and course correcting, hundreds of thousands of dollars in fuel and resources would be wasted, and surely raising frustration levels as they zigzag their way to the final destination (if they ever make it).

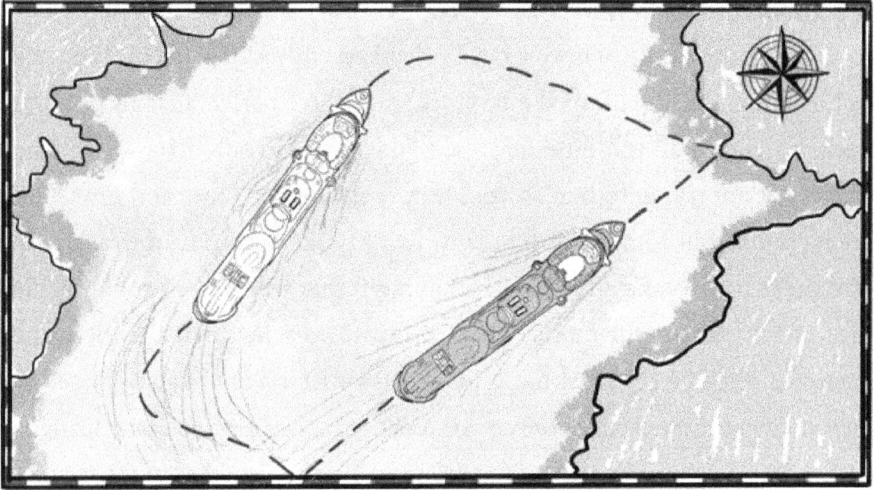

With blood sugar management strategies, if we're only checking once every three months at our quarterly check-in with our endocrinologist or doctor, we're forced to make massive adjustments in the course, often losing out on money, health, and time. But what if—and hear me out—what if we gathered blood sugar data on a more consistent basis, similar to the way a cruise ship might complete its journey? What if we did little check-ins of our own on a weekly or even daily basis for 15 minutes? How much faster (and safer) do you think we'd hit our goals? What if small, consistent adjustments and adaptations to our insulin ratios, blood sugar formulas, and lifestyle choices *were* the answer to an easier life with diabetes? If that were all it took—small "how are the blood sugars looking today" check-ins—to finally remove the mystery and frustration from living with diabetes… would it be worth it to focus your efforts for 15 minutes if you could see actual progress with blood sugar management from all the effort you're already putting in?

*****

It's All About the Data

"Bring the data, not the drama," a client recently said while on a coaching call with me. I nearly jumped out of my seat at how perfect his phrasing was. I tell my clients all the time that there is no failure, only data. Your blood sugars are not trying to punish you; they're giving you clues and hints like a breadcrumb trail for you to follow to identify the source of the issue. Any mistake that we make and learn from is a gift that will help us avoid making the same mistake in the future. That being said, mistakes that are not learned from will often be repeated until the necessary lesson is learned. "What gets measured gets managed" is only as true as the actions that you take using the data that you collect. If you notice a trend of high blood sugar in the morning but do nothing to fix it, then you will continue to have high blood sugar in the mornings until the pain of remaining the same is greater than the pain of effort and change. So gather the information, learn from your own mistakes, and whenever possible, learn from the mistakes of others.

66 ─────────────────────────

...mistakes that are not learned from will often be repeated until the necessary lesson is learned.

───────────────────────── 99

One of the greatest shortcuts in life is to use the lessons that someone else had to learn the hard way as stepping stones on your own path to speed up your progress. This is what coaches, mentors, and experts are all about—giving you the answers that they had to learn through trial and error (often over many years or even decades of their own time and efforts). This has been the greatest "life hack" I've discovered so far in my own life. When I want to learn or master something new, I find someone who's already done it successfully, and I hire them for their expert insight and accountability.

The more data that you collect, the more informed your decisions will be. It might not be a realistic long-term option for most people to track every detail every day, especially at the level of detail that diabetes requires, but I need you to commit to consistently tracking the variables that are important to you for the duration of this book. Doing so will enable you, by the end of this book, to have the metrics you need to make progress, ensuring that you're on the right path and maintaining momentum every day. You'll have patterns to look for. You'll have progress to be proud of. How much progress? It depends entirely on how driven and determined you are. Most of the clients that I work with for weeks, months, or even longer reach their goals at a sustainable pace with lasting results. That being said, we have had multi-day challenges and workshops where people achieve the goals that they set out to accomplish (like reaching 90% time in range with their blood sugars) in record time—five days or less—using the strategies taught in this book.

One of the first steps that we have those clients take on is to keep their routines relatively consistent (temporarily) and to track the ins and outs of everything related to blood sugar so that we can observe their habits, intakes, and the day-to-day differences and nuances that might have slid "under the radar" previously. When you do this, you might notice things that shock you. In fact, when they first track their food, most people *do* identify higher fat consumption than they had originally anticipated (just like my example from earlier). This isn't good or bad. It simply *is*. It's what you do with that information that matters. When tracking inputs, you get to decide whether they fall in line with your current goals and what you would like to see with your blood sugar, your weight management, and your health preferences. But the goal here is to *start* tracking so that you're able to make more predictable (and efficient) progress while identifying (and reducing) potential blood sugar blind spots. If you're not tracking your inputs, you're likely unaware of their dangerous impacts, which might be secretly holding you back or, worse, taking you completely off course and in the wrong direction. And it doesn't matter how fast you're going if it's taking you off course and moving you in the wrong direction.

There's something we call the **"ignorance tax"**—mistakes or obstacles to our success that continue to be a hindrance until we learn the lesson that they offer. The only way to protect yourself against this "tax" is to track and measure your inputs so that you can impact your results (outputs) intentionally. When we remove our ignorance of the mistake at hand (by becoming more aware of it), we can stop paying the "ignorance tax" (like when I identified the high fat I was unknowingly consuming for breakfast every day, I became less ignorant). In other words, "what gets measured gets managed."

The ignorance tax is like a ghost that follows you around day and night, tripping you up and making life harder than it needs to be. Ghosts are invisible, though, right? So the only way to get rid of something you can't see is to pay more attention to your surroundings and events to first become more aware of it. Maybe you see the flicker of a candle even though there's no wind in the room (hint: it was the ghost), or maybe you notice your friend's dog freaks out every time you come over (hint: it's the ghost again), or maybe you keep tripping over "nothing" (hint: yup, ghost again). With your added awareness that *something* is wrong, who are you gonna call? (The Ghostbusters!) You're going to call the experts, who are going to say, "Yup, there was a ghost making your life miserable. Now that you know about that (aka, you are no longer "ignorant" of it), all you have to do is sprinkle salt around you three times and sing Yankee Doodle (or whatever you do to get rid of ghosts). This ghost (or the missing pieces/gaps in your diabetes knowledge) will continue to haunt you *until* you become more aware of the impacts and learn about how to remove them from your life.

On the topic of paying the "ignorance tax," one of the reasons I was so shocked at my higher fat content was not only because of weight management and body composition but also because of blood sugar management. There's a strong correlation between high-fat diets and higher insulin resistance. So, when we can measure the patterns of our blood sugar alongside the patterns of other documented data points like food consumption or exercise routines, we can see which correlations serve us well and stabilize blood sugars and which do not. An increase in exercise might equal a decrease in our total daily dose of insulin, as exercise can improve our insulin sensitivity quite effectively. As I decreased my fat intake, I also saw a lowered need for insulin, and even less of a pre-bolus time required at meals. One of the best things you can do as you start to move through this book is simply to gather information, track it over a specified amount of time (for example, one week), and look for areas of progress or decline in order to identify what works and what must be changed.

We're taking this diabetes thing into our own hands.

This is the "**Renegade Way.**"

In the next chapter, I'll break down exactly what you can *do* about it starting right now to fix blood sugars for good.

Notes:

_____

_____

_____

_____

_____

_____

_____

_____

_____

_____

_____

_____

_____

_____

_____

_____

_____

CHAPTER 4

HOW I FIXED MY BLOOD SUGARS WITH FORMULAS

The **ARM framework** is a concept that we teach in one of our challenges that allows us to virtually guarantee 90% time in range (keeping blood sugars between 70-180 md/dL for 90% of the time in a 24-hour period) for anyone who follows what we teach. What gives me the right to guarantee such a wild outcome and teach on this topic? Well, personally, I've been over 90% time in range for over FIVE consecutive years while living my absolute best life (spending my days and nights 90% between the targets of 70-180 mg/dL, though as my average glucose and standard deviation reports would suggest, I prefer to aim for blood sugars to be 90-140 mg/dL… because, well, because I can and that's where I feel my best). I've also privately coached hundreds of T1D clients and thousands of others in larger T1D audiences to achieve similar targets, such as 90% or greater time in range, stellar A1C values, and more flexibility and freedom with food and exercise.

As you can imagine, I start many of our private coaching clients with this framework as a "life preserver" strategy for when their blood sugar gets crazy every once in a while. Think of it like a "**blood sugar reset button**" that allows us to "force" blood sugars to get back in range (and stay there for longer periods of time). What I'm about to share with you is the first practical step towards fixing your blood sugars that you can use and implement *today*. We've all had those days where we experienced a "blood sugar roller coaster," right? You've got a high number that you take too much insulin for (for me, it's typically either out of frustration or impatience), then you go low, consume too much candy or juice in a panic, then shoot back up to high blood sugar, and it's a never-ending sequence of events that inevitably yields frustration and sometimes even anger or anxiety (at least for me). The ARM framework is what we use to intentionally get off the blood sugar roller coaster and stay in range with healthy numbers.

Let's start with the first letter. **"A" stands for "Assess."** The first step in understanding how to fix blood sugars is to actually understand what's going on with them in the first place. We can use our CGM graphs to identify the different time frames and potential causes for the blood sugar that we see going up or down (more details on this in a few chapters; remember: I won't let you get lost while reading this book). Ultimately, the first step is to assess the situation at hand—just gather the information and review it. The best way to simplify this step is to just "get curious" about blood sugars. Ask yourself (with zero blame or emotion, remember it's only data), *What happened there? Why do I think that happened?*

The second step in the framework is the letter **"R," which stands for "Redirect."** I'll share something fun (and life-changing) in Chapter 6 that we call "**balancing arrows**," where we not only identify what went wrong but also learn about the actions that can be taken to remedy the situation and get us back into a stable and healthy blood sugar... sometimes in an instant.

Finally, the third step, **"M," is to "Map it out."** When we identify the root cause of the blood sugar fluctuation (Assess), and we are able to take action to bring it back in range (Redirect), we want to remember what worked and what didn't for future use. We're essentially creating a mental map or, in some cases, an actual checklist of sorts that allows us to reference these pitfalls when blood sugar doesn't cooperate. When you make it to the end of this book, I've got a surprise for you that'll bring everything together in a simple-to-understand illustration. This method allows us to remedy the situations faster (and in a safer way) in the future. For example, I used to take insulin for food or correction doses before I went for a run, and it often led me into urgent low blood sugar. I followed the ARM framework to make a better plan, which was ultimately redesigned into what is now called the **"Renegade Reset Blood Sugar Formula"** (for its ability to "reset" chaotic blood sugars). Here's a visual:

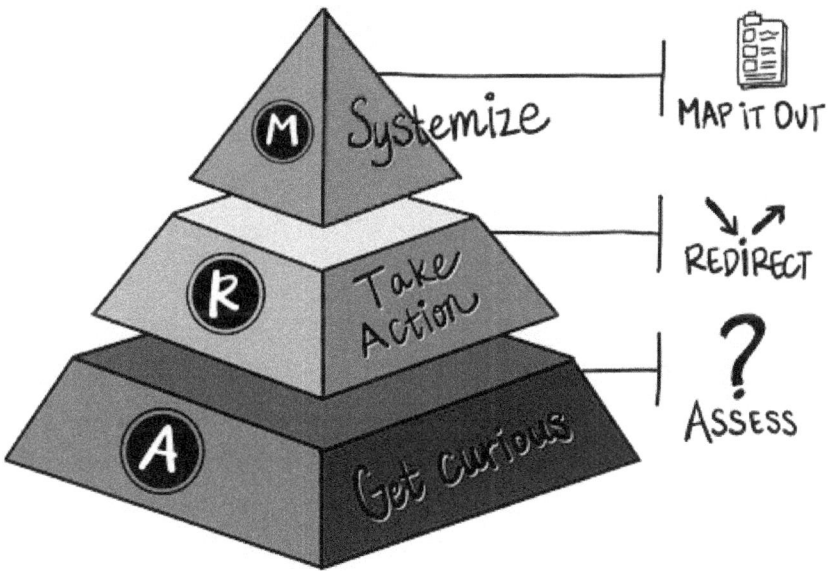

We teach this specific formula (and the ARM framework specifically) in a five-day challenge called **"The Blood Sugar Formula Challenge."** We spend a day on *each* of those steps, which allows us to go a lot more in-depth and walk you through everything. In the past, we've charged people for this experience, but because you're here with me and committed to this process, I want to give it to you for *free*. For your exclusive invite and a "reader's bundle" of resources that'll help you as you make your way through this book, SCAN THE QR CODE

Blood Sugar Formulas

Now that I've brought it up, what is a blood sugar formula, and how can it help you? Believe it or not, you've actually already been using blood sugar formulas since day one of your diagnosis. Think about it: an insulin-to-carb ratio is an equation that you use daily (or should be using) when deciding how many units of insulin you take for the carbohydrates that you consume. A similar concept (if your medical team is a little behind) is the exchange system, where you take "x" amount of insulin per serving of carbohydrate. Similar idea, but far less accurate. The real issue overall is that the formulas we've been given as diabetics are all incomplete by nature.

The definition of the word *formula* that I found online is "a mathematical relationship or rule expressed in symbols."[1] The issue with diabetes, though, is that we're not just talking about math here—we're talking about science and lifestyle factors as well. So, we define a blood sugar formula as "the organization of known and unknown variables to identify solutions and balance points." Simply put, this concept is a lot like solving a puzzle. You have some pieces that you already know where they go based on the pictures from the puzzle

---

[1] Google, s.v. "formula," accessed 2024.

box or edge pieces that you find (known variables), and some you don't quite know just yet where they go, like the sky or single-color pieces (these would be the unknown variables). In order to figure out where they connect (like looking for the solution or balance point for a blood sugar "problem"), we can look at the *context* (or the surrounding known variables), like the nearby pieces and the box they came in, to see the whole picture and give us a reference point for where things might fit together.

Heck, even if you don't have the box picture or any pieces solved, just trying to fit pieces together might land you a few lucky guesses and connection points (this is how I personally identified the pre-bolus formula—we'll call it trial and error with quite a few highs and lows until I figured it out). That being said, there are many different types of blood sugar formulas, though only a few are generic in nature. Most of them must be customized for the individual's variables and goals (which is why some people like to work with me directly to get a more personalized approach for faster and more predictable results).

Let's start with the more generic blood sugar formulas first and lay the foundation. What I'd like to do is simplify what a blood sugar formula looks like by giving you a few examples. And as I mentioned, there are many different formulas for different outcomes (think lifestyles and goals). Most formulas must be customized to fit an individual's goals (if you want to lose weight, be a professional athlete, have flexibility in the foods that you eat as you travel to beautiful locations, start a family, and so on). Let's jump in.

Decision-Making Formula

The first type I'd like to discuss is the "decision-making formula." This can be simplified into a statement of *if, then, unless.* What's interesting is that our medical teams have been using the *if-then* portion of the formula all along. They'll say, "*If* blood sugars are high, *then* you must take more insulin." The issue is that there is zero *context* being considered, which is why we added the word *unless* to the end. An example of *if-then-unless* might read, "*If* blood sugars are high, *then* I take insulin *unless* my blood sugar is already dropping rapidly." (Am I 200 mg/dL and stable, or am I 200 mg/dL and dropping fast?) Here's another one: "*If* blood sugars are high, *then* I take insulin *unless* exercise is anticipated" (which may lower blood sugar independently). From a scary experience in my own life—and you may have seen this in yours as well—I have noticed that exercise, by itself, can also lower blood sugar.

So, if I were to take insulin for high blood sugar and also exercise, then I have *two* variables that will drop my blood sugar (and they might drop too far into hypoglycemia). *If-then* can be categorized as generic advice from our medical teams, but adding the *unless* serves to convert it to a dynamic approach to represent real-life scenarios (and to improve our outcomes with blood sugar control). It allows us to add *context* to our decision-making frameworks, which in turn allows for better outcomes overall to avoid potential pitfalls or dangerous situations before they happen. This is what we teach at FTF Warrior (my type 1 diabetes education and coaching company).

Conversely, If we existed in a vacuum that's void of spontaneity and fun, where nothing changes day to day, then the *if-then* method would likely work well enough. If it were really as simple as "take insulin for high blood sugars and eat sugar for low blood sugars" (hint: it's *not* that simple), then you probably wouldn't need much more than just visiting the doctor once a year for a check up and an update on your prescriptions. Most of us don't live the exact same day over and over and over again, though (thankfully, that'd be pretty boring). As such, it's critical that we add the word *unless* to our decision-making process to cover the subtle nuances of diabetes management. If life looks different from day to day, so must our strategies.

These decision-making formulas were built for real-time adjustments using known data sets. I have to be aware of these known variables in order to know how that added *context* might influence my decision. I have to be aware of my plans to exercise and be aware of what else might be impacting blood sugar. If I don't know what to expect from exercise —whether it drops or spikes my blood sugar, or does anything at all—then I'm unable to use this formula to its full potential. Study up and observe your patterns to gain the full benefit (in other words, keep reading this book) and become more aware of your variables and impacts.

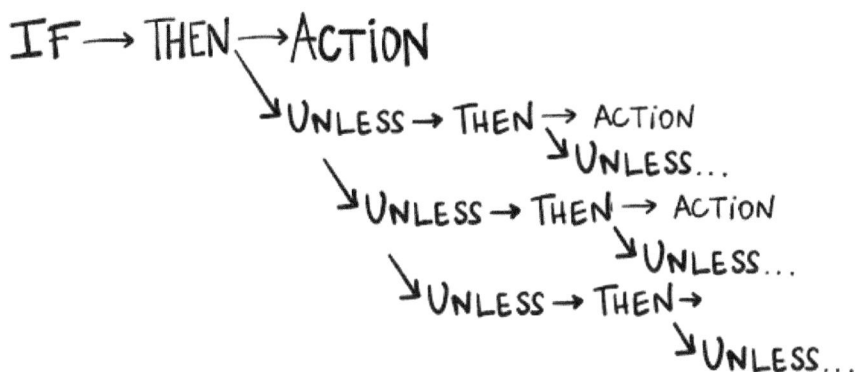

IF → THEN → ACTION
　　　↘ UNLESS → THEN → ACTION
　　　　　　　　↘ UNLESS...
　　　　↘ UNLESS → THEN → ACTION
　　　　　　　　↘ UNLESS...
　　　　↘ UNLESS → THEN →
　　　　　　　↘ UNLESS...

Solution-Finding Formula

The second formula type that I want to simplify for you is called the "**solution-finding formula**," which can be expressed as A +/- B = C. A different way to think about this formula is like a recipe to create a meal. Since I'm eating a lot of pancakes right now (because I enjoy them and know how to keep blood sugar stable through any meal), I want to use pancake mix as an example. In this example, we're "solving" for pancakes; we're trying to figure out how to end up with a fluffy, golden-brown breakfast cake. If I use one cup of water plus one cup of pancake mix, it equals a pancake.

Obviously, recipes can get more complicated, as does diabetes in many scenarios, where you might have something crazier like A + B – (C + D) = E (like trying to take insulin for pizza and maintain stable and in-range blood sugars—ha-ha), but for the sake of simplicity in this example, we are combining two known variables (pancake ingredients and water) to achieve a desired end result of a pancake. For all my math whiz friends out there looking for a written out example, we could also imagine a made-up equation where

A equals 1 and C equals negative 3; you'd be able to solve for B (which would read as 1 + B = -3, solved to be -4 in this made-up example). These solution-finding formulas were built to solve for unknown data sets as well as **"renegade resets,"** which you'll learn more about in the next few chapters of this book.

That being said, let's finish the real-life example to wrap this one up. If I want a pancake, and I know that water and pancake mix are the only ingredients needed, then it just becomes an experiment to see where the balancing point (or ratio) is for water to pancake mix. I might make a few mistakes along the way and add too much water, resulting in runny pancake batter, but with enough determination and diligence, I'd eventually figure out that the perfect pancake recipe balances at one part water, one part mix.

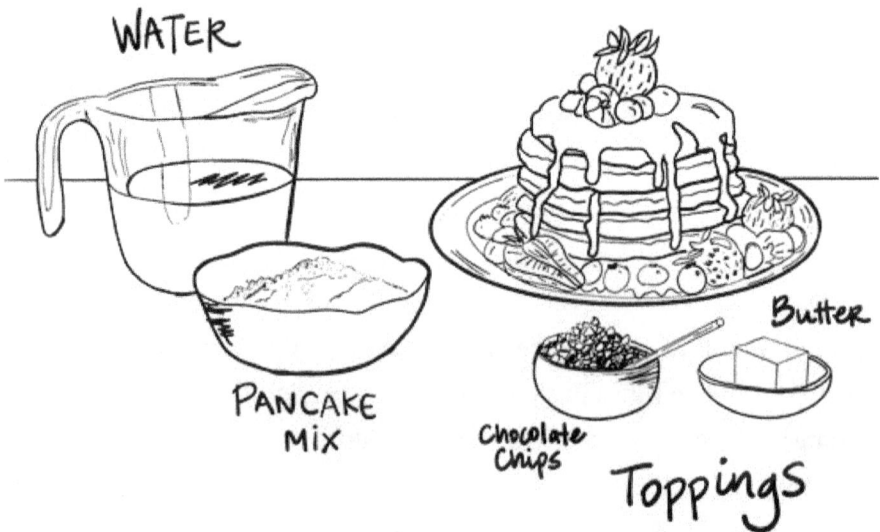

WATER

PANCAKE MIX

Chocolate Chips

Butter

Toppings

Let's explore this example through the lens of insulin-dependent diabetes. If I wanted to know what my insulin to carbohydrate ratio was, I could use this formula to accomplish just that. My goal would be to identify how many carbs (short for carbohydrates) I could eat in order to balance out the impact of 1 unit of insulin. In the bigger picture, knowing my balancing point, or "insulin-to-carb ratio," would give me more flexibility in my food choices (especially in the volume I consume them in if I were extra hungry) because I would have more certainty in how much insulin to take for any given amount of carbohydrates.

For the experiment, I might eat 20 grams of carbohydrates and take 1 unit of insulin, noting that I ended up with a high blood sugar later on. Ok, not enough insulin (because I ended up with a high blood sugar). I might try again later with 10 carbs with 1 unit of insulin and wind up with a low blood sugar. Hmm, too much insulin and not enough food. 15 carbs and 1 unit of insulin, blood sugars stayed perfectly in range—BINGO! I've essentially found my insulin-to-carb ratio (this is over-simplified, but hopefully you get the idea). Ultimately, we're looking for the balancing point with all of these equations. Now, obviously, there are *many* other variables and factors that impact whether or not your insulin-to-carb ratio is correct (including that it can change day to day - oh no!), but we'll get more to those later in this book.

In regards to the pancake example, I'm sure you're asking yourself, *Why doesn't he just check the directions on the back of the box to get the instructions on how much water to add to the pancake mix?* And that's an excellent question! *That* is what it's like to hire a coach or a mentor who can guide you through these blood sugar formulas and customize them to your liking. So instead of just memorizing the equation for *one* situation and repeating the same boring day forever, you might enjoy more flexibility and adaptability, like how the pancake recipe changes if I'm making chocolate-chip banana pancakes for my two-year-old daughter instead of "standard" pancakes.

I'm sure you're now saying to yourself, *Great, but "diabetes math" sounds pretty complicated...*

I'll say it again because I know it can sound scary - I promise you that if you can do simple addition and subtraction (like 1 + 1 = 2), then you're gonna love this formula method. If you can't do basic math, put this book down and buy a calculator that can do the math for you before going any further (problem solved).

In the example above, we solved for the pancake with the formula because it allowed me to organize and identify what was needed and in what ratio to achieve a desired result (the delicious pancake). So, if I wanted, for example, to eat a pancake as a diabetic, I would want to know how much insulin is required for that food and when I need to take that insulin to time the dose correctly. The *context* from our "decision-making formula" would be identifying current blood sugars, what my insulin on board is, if there was any planned activity after the meal, and so on. But the idea is that if I wanted to achieve stable blood sugar when eating a pancake, I'd have to know what the recipe for success in that circumstance looks like. If I want to know what's needed to keep blood sugar stable during a long run, I need to know how many carbs I need to consume to offset the drop that I expect from the activity of running, and I also might want to consider any adjustments to my insulin. I'm building and collecting these formulas as I go to achieve a specific and desired outcome (one that looks different for all of us).

These "**solution-finding formulas**" were built to solve unknown data sets where I know what I want (like eating a pancake or determining an insulin-to-carb ratio), but I don't yet know exactly what strategy to use to get there. I have to use my thinking brain to identify what's necessary for blood sugar control so I can take action to accomplish stable blood sugar with that desired solution. We also call these our "**renegade resets**" in our "**Blood Sugar Formula Challenge**" because when blood sugars are chaotic, finding a quick *solution* to balance them out can be incredibly helpful - for our health, but also for our sanity. Hence the term: "**solution-finding formula.**"

In fact, when blood sugar is absolutely chaotic for me (yes, that happens to me as well from time to time), I need to know how to reset it to get off the "blood sugar roller coaster." Sometimes, the strategy will look a little bit different from what we were taught in our doctor's office, which is why we call them our "**renegade resets.**" As "**renegade warriors,**" we *think differently.* We don't only think in terms of insulin or sugar. We look at the whole picture and consider our options. We don't wait until we're urgently low to treat low blood sugar like we were taught in our doctor's office (remember the "rule of 15" from earlier). Heck, I might micro-treat with small amounts of sugar before I even get into a low blood sugar to avoid this situation entirely (especially if there is activity planned, insulin on board, or if I can *see* on a CGM that I'm headed toward a low in the near future). This is something we teach in our online challenge as well (that you have free access to as my gift to you for grabbing this book—scan the QR code at the beginning or end of the book to access).

*****

Predictive Planning Formula

Now, my personal favorite is the "**predictive planning formula.**" An example of this would be the "**80/20 Blood Sugar Formula**" that I use in my own life and has allowed me to maintain above 90% of the time in range for the last 5+ years straight since implementing it, all while living my life to the fullest, training for triathlon and Ironman races, traveling and eating all the fun and delicious foods, and even running around like crazy as a business owner and parent. It's also what I teach my private T1D clients so that they can live their best lives as well. That being said, this formula can only be effectively used when it's customized to the individual. We all have different goals, struggles, and diabetes variables to consider, and it would be irresponsible for me to pretend there's some cookie-cutter approach that's the exact same for everyone. Because it's a customized formula, the only place to set this up for your personal needs is to work with me and my team directly.

For example, I know from my own blood sugar formula that if I want to go for an hour mountain bike ride by myself in the middle of nowhere, I need 11 to 12 grams of complex carbs per 30 minutes of activity in order to keep me perfectly stable between 90 and 110 mg/dL. But for my Ironman training bike rides (60-100 miles at a time), I need more than triple that rate (300+

carbs for my last ride, around 60-90 carbs per hour depending on intensity) to stay in range (which is kinda nice, honestly—you get super hungry when you're four or five hours into a workout). Keep in mind this is for *me* and my needs. Without the formula, I'd have probably landed in the hospital (or worse) on multiple occasions because it would have been a guessing game. These formulas are what enable me to feel and act "normal" again, and they've given me my quality of life and peace of mind back as well. I'll also note (because I know it's a question asked by many) that you do *not* have to be an elite athlete in order to qualify to work with me. I am, in fact, kinda crazy with this whole Ironman kick I've been on recently. In fact, most of my clients are just trying to live their day-to-day lives with less blood sugar stress, spend more time with loved ones, and feel "normal" again with healthy blood sugars that don't require them to "babysit" their diabetes.

The ultimate goal of this predictive method is to give you the opportunity to keep blood sugar stable through a specific exercise or a fun meal (or even just day-to-day living, as I mentioned above) by knowing what's necessary as an exchange or balance point to keep blood sugars exactly where you want them. Alternatively, you can also predict where blood sugar is going to go using this method as well. If that predicted blood sugar is undesirable, you need to know exactly which actions to take—or not take—in order to *manipulate* blood sugars to end up where you want them to be. *That* is the power of blood sugar formulas—taking back the power to control blood sugar so that the blood sugar doesn't control you. We'll get more into manipulating blood sugars at will in Chapter 6 as well, and yes, it's as fun and exciting as it sounds. For now, I want you to think of the different "pieces" of type 1 diabetes formulas like building blocks that stack on top of each other. The more you learn, the further you go, the easier it gets.

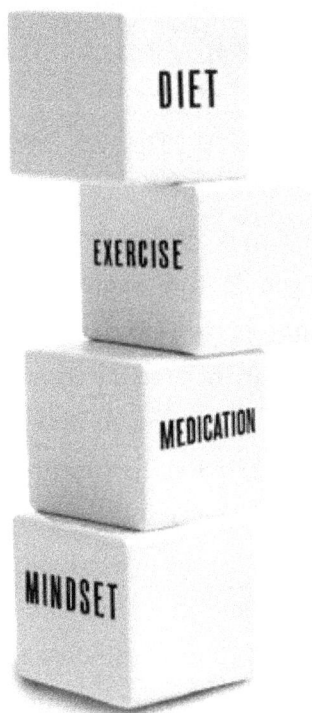

As you've read about blood sugar formulas so far, you might already be saying to yourself, *Oh, I think I already have some blood sugar formulas in place. You know, my doctor gave me an insulin-to-carb ratio, or insulin sensitivity factor, or the rule of 15 for lows.* This is true in part, but the issue is that they are incomplete formulas, which can be detrimental to your health and even pose potential threats to your life. In fact, there was this one time that my doctor and my endo both told me—as they've most likely told many of you—that I need to take my insulin 10 to 15 minutes before my meals, *no matter what.* This is called a "pre-bolus," which allows your insulin time to work before a meal, with the goal of achieving more stable blood sugar and avoiding a post-meal spike.

If this seems new to you, and to break down the reason we might consider this strategy, I'll give you an example before detailing why it's a broken and outdated method. I want you to imagine that insulin and your meal are two different people who are going to go to a party. They live at different locations that are different distances from the destination where the party is being held.

Insulin calls up food and says, "Hey, are you going to the party at nine?" Food says, "Heck yes, I'll be there."

Insulin responds, "Okay, great. Since you live closer than I do, I need to leave 15 minutes before you do if we want to arrive at the party at the same time together." Because no one wants to go to a party and not know anybody. It's embarrassing and awkward to sit in the corner alone, waiting for friends.

So, Insulin says, "Hey, I'm going to leave now, and you leave in 15 minutes, and that way, we'll arrive at the same time."

Fifteen minutes later, food takes off, and insulin and food arrive at the party at the same time, and everyone lived happily ever after.

This is the desired outcome for a pre-bolus. For most of our fast-acting insulins today, it takes about 10 to 15 minutes to start working. Food has a near-instantaneous impact (it lives right next door to the party) as it begins immediately breaking down in our mouth once we take a bite and continues to break down and impact blood sugars as it travels through our gastrointestinal tract (digestive system). We have to time our insulin and food properly in order to achieve stable blood sugar after a meal, hence this "rule" or formula that many of us were given of the 15-minute pre-bolus. The issue with that is that these rules we're given in the endo's office are static. They do not apply to every area of our life because diabetes changes day to day, minute to minute. Situational awareness, or *context*, is critical. Our strategies need to be dynamic because no two days (or meals) are truly identical, even if you eat the same food.

For example, if I start a meal with a blood sugar of 60 mg/dL and I'm currently going low, do I want my blood sugar to stay low (or worse, be at risk of going lower)? The answer is no. So, using that context of *if-then-unless* in this situation, I would decide that *if* I'm about to eat, *then* I take my insulin 15 minutes early, *unless* I'm already low. Then, I would make a new decision to either reduce or remove the pre-bolus and consider reducing or removing my bolus if I wanted to get blood sugar back to a healthy spot that was not dangerous.

Another example is the type of food (and I could go on for *days* with different examples of things that impact pre-bolus timing). If I'm eating a fruit smoothie, that's likely to hit my blood sugar a lot faster than something slower digesting, like a veggie omelet. Something that impacts blood sugars faster might need a longer pre-bolus time, whereas something slow digesting might not need a pre-bolus at all. Nutrition is a deep topic, and this is only scratching the surface, but hopefully, this is sparking some "ah-ha" moments for you as to why your efforts and strategies might not have been working before you read this book. Read on for more lightbulb moments.

Just like the pre-bolus rule of taking insulin 10 to 15 minutes before eating no matter what, these incomplete formulas and rules that surround us do not always apply. They provide a helpful starting point, but we need more precision if we expect to have any hope of living healthy and happy lives that aren't constantly interrupted by diabetes. It falls on our shoulders as **"renegade warriors"** to *think differently* about how we can navigate these unique situations because daily life with diabetes does not exist in a vacuum (without change or interruptions). It is not consistent. Life is chaotic and wonderful and adventurous. As such, our strategies have to be able to adapt. So, when we think about formulas, I want you to understand that formulas allow us to adapt to different situations. They give us the power to change our approach when the strategies we've been given don't line up with our current circumstances.

*****

The "Best Guess" Advice

When we're told to pre-bolus early by our medical teams (hopefully, they're at least telling you about the pre-bolus, though I hear horror stories often of medical teams that are completely incompetent), we have to take a more dynamic approach with the whole picture in mind. We need to consider outside variables that might change the rules that diabetes is playing by *on that day*. For example, do I have recent insulin on board that might affect my total dose for this meal? Or have I exercised recently, which would impact my insulin sensitivity (potentially lowering the amount of insulin I need overall)? These are factors that would change how much insulin I take and when I take it. And if I'm ignorant of these or told that they don't matter, I put myself in a position where I could be at risk of going into an urgent low or extreme high, leaving me feeling hopeless and frustrated that diabetes defeated me again.

Another example of this might be your insulin-to-carb ratio, which, by the way, is your doctor's "best guess" at how much insulin you should be taking on day one. The reality is that they don't know with full certainty how much insulin you need. It's their "best guess," and that's why they tell you to let them know how it goes after you give it a few tries. How terrifying is it to know that we're playing with a medication that could save us or kill us with just a few units difference if gone unchecked? They're telling you to guess on your medication and report back, which should be the first sign that we are indeed our own best doctors from day one.

The insulin-to-carb ratio is their "best guess" at telling you how much insulin you need for the carbohydrates you consume. What they don't tell you, though, is that **we also have to consider insulin-to-protein**. Yes, I said it; there is insulin that must be taken for protein, but the *timing* and the *volume* are going to differ depending on the *context* of the situation. There's that word again, *context*. We'll get to this later, but you might also consider your fat content when making dosing decisions. High-fat foods can slow down the absorption of carbs, which can assist in reducing an after-meal blood sugar spike initially, but excess consumption of fat can also lead to higher levels of insulin resistance or a plateaued high blood sugar after a meal (even hours later).

All in all, when we consider insulin-to-protein or insulin-to-fat resistance, I recall the example I gave earlier where my endo back in the day ended up bumping up my basal insulin for years on end, thinking that *if* blood sugars are high, *then* give more insulin, but it was the higher fats and proteins from my meals that were jacking up my blood sugar all along. This happens with a lot of my clients as well because endocrinologists and doctors see high blood sugar and think *more insulin*, but all they're doing is just treating the symptoms instead of searching for the root cause. They put Band-Aid fixes on us year after year after year, which only leads to compounding "below-the-surface" problems later on. In the case of a few clients of mine, it led to their medical teams setting their basal insulin to more than twice the amount they needed while still adding more and more and more to try to fix the surface-level issues (post-meal blood sugar spikes), when all they needed was a longer pre-bolus or a stronger insulin-to-carb ratio. This "mislabeling" of the root cause is more common than you might think.

In fact, I remember a client of mine who had told me after going through our program that he needed help with exactly this. It was only after finally getting his insulin ratios dialed in while working with us that he discovered he had been consuming an enormous number of calories just to avoid going low because of the poor decisions that his medical team had made in the absence of *context*. They noticed a pattern of delayed high blood sugars after meals and had him taking *twice* as much basal insulin as he actually needed in an attempt to remedy that struggle. No wonder he was having such difficulty controlling blood sugar before our program! In addition to that, once we fixed the root cause to keep blood sugar in control, he didn't have to "feed" the extra insulin throughout the day in an effort to avoid lows, and he watched the pounds drop from his belly weight that he'd been helplessly trying (and failing) to lose for *years* before choosing to work with us.

When we have *context*—like higher blood sugar might actually be due to a higher protein meal (and not necessarily a lack of proper basal insulin)—then instead of solving for something generic like high blood sugar, we can solve for the root cause, like the meal itself, and look at the unknown variables we might consider solving for instead. This is where **"cause and effect"** comes into play. One of my favorite discussions with clients is to respond to a theory they have on why blood sugar is high or low with a chat on "correlation versus causation." Is my high blood sugar directly caused by something I ate, or is it simply a correlation with this variable, and the root cause is something else?

Another one of my clients I chatted with had a theory that drinking fruit juice caused lower blood sugar for her. She had tracked her blood sugar, and every time she had juice, her sugar would go down. Of course, this raised some questions for me as her coach because the effect of juice is typically a higher, not a lower, blood sugar. However, as we dug into the situational details (the *context*), we found out that the juice was often what she was using to rehydrate during and after exercising. So it wasn't necessarily the juice causing the low, but rather, the exercise that she had just completed that had actually caused the drop in blood sugar. The juice was masking it because she attributed it to the wrong variable since multiple variables were at play.

This is what we call **"mislabeling,"** and it can be extremely dangerous. If she continued thinking that juice lowered her blood sugar and decided to drink it when her blood sugar was high, she could end up in the hospital with DKA (diabetic ketoacidosis) or worse. Believe it or not, there is a good chance that you've mislabeled the effects of different blood sugar variables out of ignorance (because diabetes is *so* complex, and we don't have the help from our medical system to interpret all of this data, so we need to put all the pieces together ourselves). We'll cover this later in the book in more detail, but the more we can isolate variables (like when I had my client go for a walk without drinking juice to see what happens from *just* walking), the easier it will be to spot true causation instead of worrying about correlation misleading you.

One of the more popular variables (and difficult to master), is to look at our insulin-to-carb ratio (how much insulin you take when you eat a meal) to identify whether or not it might be working. It's important to note that this is also an incomplete formula because in addition to your insulin-to-carb ratio, you need to have your insulin-to-protein ratio, your insulin-to-fat resistance ratio, *and* your basal rates dialed in, And this assumes you have the rest of your 50+ variables perfected as well so that there's nothing else potentially acting on blood sugars during your meal time (like added insulin resistance or insulin sensitivity for the day). I know it sounds like a lot, and it is, but reading through this book and going through the additional resources it comes with will help you put together all of these pieces with more clarity. Don't give up. Keep reading!

*****

Solving the Puzzle

Once you start to pick up a little momentum, the fun part is to recognize that these different formulas all fit together like puzzle pieces, and you'll see that the big picture is incredibly simple when it's all set up. And as we'll discuss later in this book, these formulas can be simplified into something that's more predictive for tight control or set on auto-pilot for less effort and more freedom and spontaneity, depending on what *you're* looking to gain from blood sugar formulas. For me, this journey stemmed from an obsession to control blood sugars that was initially very unhealthy and desperate but later turned into a blend of happy and healthy when I was able to maintain control over my blood sugar *while* living my life to the fullest.

At the start of my journey, my desire to learn came from needing to know why I almost died multiple times; it was survival instinct masked as curiosity. My doctor didn't help, my endocrinologist couldn't satisfy my desire for a thriving life with T1D and told me, "That's just how diabetes is," and, as someone who prefers being proactive instead of waiting until it's too late, the medical system as a whole was too complacent for my taste. So, I needed to solve for an unknown variable set (stable and predictable blood sugars), and my journey to discover the first-ever blood sugar formula began out of sheer desperation.

To be completely transparent, I was a broken human at that point in my life. My quality of life was horrendous. I questioned if life was even worth living at one point as I struggled to make it through everyday tasks. Just eating a meal and doing the dishes had me filled with fears of lows and highs and hospital trips. I was terrified for things to go wrong again with my blood sugars, so wrong that I might not make it through this time. And these unknowns pushed me to dive headfirst into research with a *do-or-die* mentality. If this hadn't worked, I don't know that I'd still be here today. Freedom with blood sugar was what I was after, and it's one of the main reasons that formulas were born.

I find that there are often **two big problems that formulas solve** for diabetics like me. Sometimes it's just one of them, but for me, it was both.

The first one is that formulas give us more predictability and certainty with control over blood sugar. If you set up your blood sugar formula properly, and I teach you the basics of that in this book, you will have more stable blood sugar as a result. Period. And while being able to say "I'm going to eat this meal and end with my blood sugars at 120 mg/dL" with confidence is exciting, you'll also have a better understanding of how to keep it more consistently stable and in range when life gets more chaotic as well. This first step is most helpful for those experiencing unpredictable and difficult-to-manage blood sugars, often feeling like diabetes "can't be controlled," and just looking for more stability and consistency overall.

The second problem that formulas fix—and it took me a few years to realize I needed this—is the ability to have more quality of life and peace of mind with flexibility and freedom. It's kinda like "cruise control" with diabetes, where you still have to keep your hands on the wheel of the car, but you're able to think about it less and actually enjoy the ride more. From my own experiences, initially, I just needed to know that my blood sugar would be stable without risking random spikes and drops. I wanted to reduce the anxiety and daily panic attacks I was having. All I cared about was having more (or any) certainty and confidence in my numbers, and I didn't care if I had to eat cardboard for the rest of my life if that's what it took. The second step is more for those seeking an auto-pilot approach—people who already have decent control but feel like too much effort or attention is required (constantly "babysitting" their diabetes) or feel restricted by food, activity, and fun as the only options to keep things stable. They look good "on paper" but want to experience more freedom while thriving with diabetes.

During my research phase, I was so sick of mysterious fluctuations. My blood sugar seemed to have a mind of its own. I felt like I was living in a madhouse, and I had no idea if or why things were going up or down all the time. The generic formulas previously mentioned solved that for me. Consistency, predictability, stability. But then, after a couple of years, I realized I had restricted myself by becoming dependent on routine, and I was saying no to all of the fun things in life. My quality of life had suffered tremendously as I had essentially built a "diabetes prison" around myself to keep my blood sugar happy. I felt depressed when I realized how much I was missing out on and how much effort it took to introduce *any* level of spontaneity or fun. I had sacrificed my quality of life in order to build stable blood sugar, living *for* my diabetes instead of *with* my diabetes.

Maybe that doesn't resonate with you. Maybe you fall more into category number two, where formulas are beneficial for you because your blood sugar is already controlled "good enough," but it takes a lot of energy to do it. Maybe it sometimes feels like all we *can* do is add more effort, more discipline, more consistency, and more restriction to keep the blood sugar happy. But the reality is that with the right blood sugar formula, you can have so much certainty in your numbers and predictability built in that you're able to lift up your head and look around at what else you want from life. You're able to spend more time with family, as I have with my own. You're able to travel without worrying about the "what ifs" so often. You're able to enjoy the food that you want to eat. And because blood sugar is so well controlled, you're able to finally feel that sense of freedom you felt before you were diagnosed with diabetes. It almost gives us back a sense of "normalcy."

Formulas give both confidence and certainty in controlled blood sugar, but they also give us the ability to enjoy more of life *because* blood sugar becomes predictable, and we can worry about it less. In fact, my mental health is finally making a comeback from things as serious as depression and suicidal thoughts after that Paris incident, where I experienced the deepest, darkest moments of my entire life. At that time, my blood sugar demanded my full attention, and it ruled every waking moment. I needed certainty for my own peace of mind. Once I had that peace of mind from logical control (through restriction and consistency), I was able to lean on my blood sugar formulas and put my diabetes into more of a "cruise control" style of management, which is where I've remained to this day. *Control comes first, and Freedom follows shortly thereafter.*

Then, of course, as I mentioned, after gaining that near-perfect control where I had flat blood sugar that was stable and predictable and beautiful on paper, that's when I realized I was only getting that result because of severe restriction and a lot of effort put in. A lot of people get stuck at this point because they fear losing the control that they worked so hard to gain; I was there, too. In fact, it got to a low point where 90% of dinner table discussions with my wife and family were about blood sugar: what I learned that day, what I didn't know, why it happened, and the frustrations that I experienced.

One day, my wife pulled me aside and told me she wanted to be supportive but didn't know how because all I ever talked about was diabetes, and she was getting a bit overwhelmed by it all. She's incredibly supportive—more than most, from what I hear—and it was getting to the point where I was being a burden, even for her. It's amazing to me that she endured that phase of my life because I was a neurotic nightmare to deal with (and that's putting it lightly).

The issue is that for many of us out there, more effort focused on our diabetes is all we know as a "strategy." We're told to document blood sugars and look for patterns, but without the root cause or blood sugar formulas to help us *interpret* that data, we get stuck in the insanity cycle - where we keep doing more of the same thing, expecting different results. The true problem is that with diabetes, more effort and restriction actually work to a certain extent, giving us this false confidence that it's going to keep working and we should keep doing it. But in the long term this strategy leads to poor quality of life and burnout while never yielding anything more than pseudo-control, at least in my experience. Trying harder with the wrong strategy can only get you so far.

*****

Understanding the Unknown Variables

During that phase of my life, where I realized that I needed to break free from the restrictive "diabetes prison" I had built for myself, I began to experiment and solve for these unknown variables, ultimately developing a revolutionary new framework for managing this beast of a disease that nearly took my life on multiple occasions. I want you to understand, and I want to drive this point home: **formulas are the only way to have both a happy *and* healthy life with type 1 diabetes**. See, often you can have a happy life like I did when I was "**stupid fearless**," ignored my diabetes, and did whatever I wanted while pretending it didn't slow me down. I took care of myself "good enough," but not quite as well as I should have.

Conversely, a lot of people will choose to live in restriction to be healthy because they want to be here for a long period of time. They restrict themselves to low-carb, keto, vegan, or other diets with lots of rules and regulations. They say no to family and friends' events. They avoid doing fun things if they have too much insulin on board or if their blood sugar isn't exactly where they want it to be. They live as a prisoner of their diabetes for the sake of control and longevity.

As I've heard from so many of my clients, they live as passengers in life while diabetes drives the car. And all they want, more than anything else, is to be back in the driver's seat and go where they want in life without diabetes dictating the route. Diabetes can be a passenger; that's fine. It's part of my life, and I know it's not going anywhere. But I refuse to give diabetes the power of decision in my life. I refuse to let it hold me back from actually living my life to the fullest.

These formulas, I understand, might sound a bit complicated, but I promise you they're truly as simple as addition and subtraction. And I'm going to show you exactly what I mean by that in the next chapter.

Notes:

_____

_____

_____

_____

_____

_____

_____

_____

_____

_____

_____

_____

_____

_____

_____

_____

CHAPTER 5

HOW TO BE YOUR OWN DOCTOR

Anytime you make a primary care or endocrinology appointment, your medical team typically has one goal: identifying what's wrong and giving their "best guess" at a solution. In this chapter, I'm going to break down their methods and give you the answers in such a simplified manner that you will be able to act as your own doctor (keep in mind that this is *not* medical advice—I can't stress that enough). The one goal they have during your 15-minute appointment can be summed up as "**pattern recognition**." They'll look over your blood sugar logs, CGM data, or whatever information you give them, which in turn gives them "ideas" for adjustments to make. This is truly a "best guess" for them because no one, literally no one, has more *context* to the numbers and blood sugar trends that you experience than you. The added frustration for us (and them) is that they often have less than 15 minutes to make all of their adjustments with whatever *context* exists in your memory from over the last three to six months.

With this in mind, what would be more ideal for me to have is the knowledge of what to look for myself. I have the *context* for each situation already in my head, and that empowers me to make the best decisions for my own diabetes management, especially if it's a recent event and not months ago (like when my endo used to ask me, "Hey, what's this random 300 mg/dL blood sugar from 2 months ago?"—as if I remember that). In this chapter, I'll teach you how to take your diabetes management into your own hands, what your doctors *should* be doing, and how to make more informed decisions than they ever could.

Back in the day, when my endo incorrectly increased my insulin at the wrong times (and for the wrong reasons), she was blind to the *context* and my day-to-day strategies, habits, and schedules, and it led her to an assumption and a mislabeling of the actual problem, which is very dangerous when playing with insulin. She noticed that I was having a rise many hours after my meals, and she assumed it was due to low basal/long-acting insulin. So when she increased my long-acting insulin, and it resulted in low blood sugar every single night, she was dumbfounded. The day-time blood sugar rises had been "fixed," but it had created a new problem with the nighttime lows: a classic game of cat and mouse.

The reality is that the high-protein and high-fat diet I was consuming at the time was leading to a delayed rise in blood sugar, which, in and of itself, is still not being talked about in many medical communities. As an expert myself, I can understand where they get lost—high protein/high fat meals DO mimic the effects of a basal rate that's too low (the effect being a "drifting" blood sugar that slowly and consistently rises up and up many hours after a meal has been finished), and it takes a trained eye to spot the difference. Instead of teaching you how to "just add more insulin" in a quick Band-Aid fix like they might, I want to show you how to identify the root cause of your blood sugar going up or down so that you know what could be causing fluctuations in the big picture and what to adjust on a more detailed level in order to achieve blood sugar that is *actually* stable.

Not too long ago, I was talking with a client (we'll call her Jennifer to protect her identity), and she was furious with her endocrinologist. After years of struggle and feeling like she was running in circles with all the effort she had been putting into her diabetes management with little to no results, she came to me with some excellent questions after seeing a few of my videos on YouTube (you can search "FTF Warrior" to find hundreds of videos there).

Jennifer mentioned that when showing her endo her CGM graphs, she was told that her blood sugar graphs looked perfect on paper, maybe even at 90 mg/dL for hours on end, but Jennifer would complain that something had to be off because it felt like it took so much effort just to keep things steady. Her endo replied with the all-too-familiar phrases, "That's just how life with diabetes is," and "You're doing better than most of my other T1D patients, don't change anything." It kills me to hear so many people being told to "settle" for a lower quality of life with type 1 diabetes because here's the thing—it does *not* have to be that hard, and you do *not* have to settle. I told her, "You tell me about all the effort that's going into keeping it steady at 90 mg/dL, but only *you* would know that you had to continually snack all day and 'feed the insulin' in order to keep it from going low. So *you* need to be the one to interpret the data, not your endo. That's what I'm here to do with you." One of my roles as a coach is to act as an "interpreter," and I'll have my clients tell me their "story" of the day so that we can identify what things actually mean (and avoid mislabeling).

Her endo, upon hearing that it was so much effort that required her to micromanage her blood sugar with snacks all day, again shrugged her shoulders and said, "It's a never-ending balancing act. Sorry, but you'll just have to deal with it."

The issue in so many of these situations is that the endo looks *only* at the numbers, not the *context*. "Numbers look good, so don't change a thing." I hear it all the time. But if the numbers look good only when the quality of life suffers, what good are the numbers in the first place? To me, that doesn't sound sustainable, which means that the "good enough" numbers aren't going to last forever… they'll only last until "diabetes burnout" shows up (which I've experienced multiple times, and it's not a pretty sight).

Something I hear quite often is that doctors will tell their patients (who later become my clients because of this) that everything "looks good" and to stop trying so hard for improvement. But these doctors don't see how much effort and attention is required to keep things "looking" stable. To top it off, whether they recognize it or not, our medical teams are comparing our "good enough" with their other patients who are "non-compliant" and suffering miserably. When they look at us, they think, *Huh, you're actually not too bad since you're not actively dying; keep up the great work!* The tough part with that is that your "good enough" is only labeled that way on paper, not in real life. Plus, if you're anything like me, I refuse to settle for anything but the best, so "good enough" is a bit of an insult. Without the *context* that you have from your daily life, no medical team can ever make as much of an informed decision as *you* can, which is why it's critical for you to gain the new strategies from this book and understand how they can help make decisions for you so that with your own empowered actions, you can start seeing improvement even outside of the doctor's office. Just promise me that you tell them about this book when their jaw hits the floor at your next visit because they can't figure out how you made such an incredible leap in blood sugar control and freedom. More people need to know what is possible; that's where you come in to help us spread the word about what you're reading here.

*****

Retrospective Analysis

Continuing a previous chapter's theme of documentation (what gets measured, gets managed) to give us this *context* for decision-making, it's helpful to review the data that we have, especially the data that our diabetes devices, like an insulin pump or a CGM, collect. In a process I want to teach you that we call "retrospective analysis" in our programs, we take a glance at the end of the day or the end of the week to see what worked, what didn't, and what might be adjusted to stabilize blood sugar moving forward. This allows us to learn from our mistakes and successes while they are still fresh in our minds, just by looking back over our day and identifying areas for improvement or changes from the information we already have. Just 15 minutes at the end of the day. That's all it takes to review your notes, ask yourself questions, ask your coach, and make progress happen instead of existing at the mercy of your diabetes and hoping it gets better. Remember, "**Nothing changes if nothing changes.**"

Let's look at an example. If you're anything like me, when you were in school and had a big exam coming up, you might have procrastinated until the night before. I often spent a few chaotic hours with energy drinks, cramming for my tests, reviewing my notes, and trying to force the topics to stay at the top of my mind in an effort to pass my test the next day. The goal, of course, was to refresh my mind on what I'd learned previously in the semester so I could recall the information needed to pass the exam, but over the years, I've learned that cramming is never as effective as small study sessions consistently repeated throughout the school year. What worked significantly better was actually going over notes each day from class and making sure that I understood the concepts, while the lessons and information from that day were still fresh in my mind. What we're talking about with this diabetes "retrospective analysis" is reviewing our notes at the end of the day while the information is still fresh so that we can make adjustments for a better tomorrow. Now, this is easiest when done with a CGM, but with enough blood sugar finger pricks (with a glucometer) and documented blood sugar numbers, it can be an effective strategy for anyone with diabetes, even without the latest technology.

Remember from earlier, "**What gets measured gets managed.**" In this chapter, we're learning about pattern recognition, and we'll cover how to analyze your CGM data, your pump data, insulin timing, blood sugar peaks, and ultimately, how to identify why your blood sugar did what it did, which is a never-ending lesson, even for me. I want you to feel confident in knowing how to proactively make changes that help you to avoid blood sugar blunders. So, step number one is to open up your CGM graph reports (or documented blood sugar logs) and observe without judging yourself. We just want to see the numbers for what they are: data. You can do this with your report from today, either on your mobile device or on a computer. If you wear a device that keeps your data for more than a week or two, it can be helpful to look at big-picture averages as well (like "Oh, I've been running higher than I typically do for the last two weeks. I wonder what changed two weeks ago that might have led to this?"). When looking at your daily graphs, I want you to **identify "problem areas."** What we're initially looking for are any spikes or drops that were either *unanticipated* or *undesired*, which allows us to consider any changes we might make for the next day.

Real-life example: I pulled up my CGM reports and noticed that I spiked from 87 mg/dL (my fasting number) up to about 150 mg/dL after breakfast this morning. Because it's fresh in my mind as I use "retrospective analysis," I can recall that I wanted to "push" my blood sugar up a little higher to give me a buffer because I had to take my daughter to a doctor's appointment and run a few errands. I wanted to be a little higher than normal so that I had a "buffer" in case I dropped while out and about. I take that as data, not as good or bad, just data. Had I waited weeks or even months to review my data, I would have NO idea why blood sugars jumped on that day. This exercise is *only* to gain information for step number two. This leads me to my secondary dive into my CGM graphs to have a look at the bigger-picture averages. It turns out I actually do have a pattern over many weeks of a similar (almost identical) spike after breakfast. I'm not as excited about that because those were less functional and likely fall under the category of "oopsie." Let's see what we can do about it.

*****

Spikes, Plateaus, Rolling Hills and Stability

The second step of this process is to identify the undesirable (or unexpected) fluctuations in blood sugars, and then we want to identify the shape on our graph.

There are four main shapes we'll be covering in this book as they relate specifically to post-meal blood sugar analysis.

The first is a **spike**, as you'll see in this drawing.

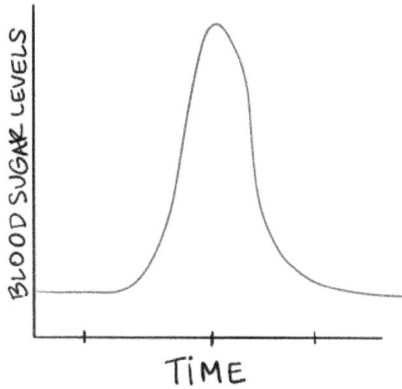

This often indicates an error in the *timing* of insulin or a consumption of fast-acting carbohydrates. In my example earlier, I saw a spike because I cut a few minutes out of my pre-bolus timing (which is when we give insulin a head start before eating food). Therefore, my issue was that of "insulin timing." More on that in a later chapter.

The second shape is a **plateau**, which can be characterized as a rise in blood sugar that gets stuck in higher numbers and may come down hours later, often after an additional dose of insulin.

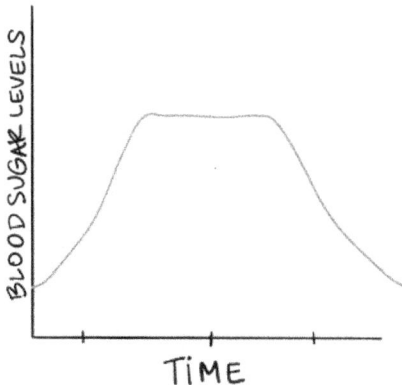

This can often be solved by better timing of the insulin (as it often occurs on the backend of a spike, or when delayed - from a protein rise), potentially revisiting the volume of insulin given (see insulin-to-carb ratio), or even considering an insulin-to-protein or insulin-to-fat-resistance ratio depending on how much of a correction dose had to be given in order to bring blood sugars back down into a healthy range.

The third shape we'll be covering is the "**rolling hills**." The small hill on a CGM graph is often indicative of a proper dose of insulin, where we see a small rise and fall of blood sugars that don't go out of range.

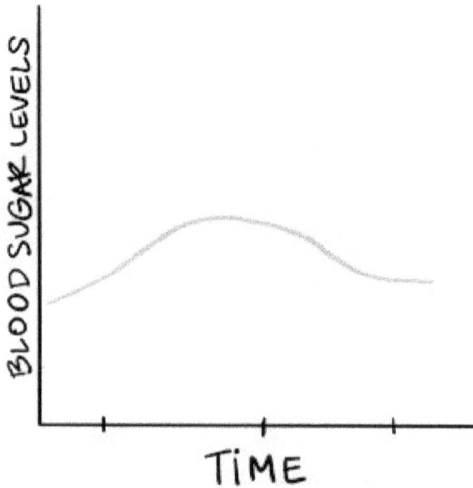

Note: Even non-diabetics see a rise in blood sugar when consuming a meal, though it's often minimal and comes back down rather quickly because of the speed of properly working insulin in a fully functioning pancreas.

The fourth, which is often overlooked, is the **stable blood sugar line**, where blood sugars have very little movement at all.

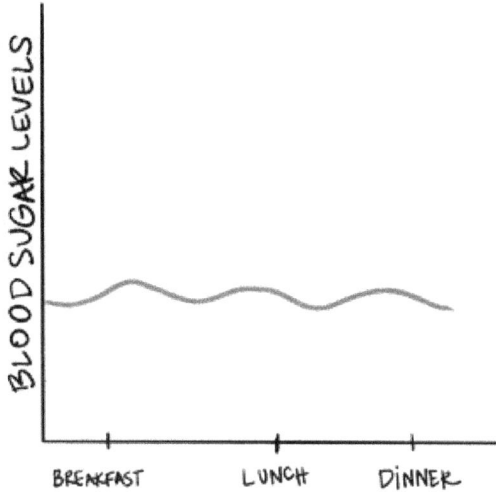

Believe it or not, because we can manipulate when our insulin is given, we technically have the potential to see *more* stable blood sugars than a non-diabetic (though it's quite difficult). I proved this in a video on our YouTube channel (search FTF Warrior on YouTube) with my wife, where I had more stable blood sugars than she did (she does not have diabetes) after eating an enormous amount of carbs (we enjoyed Chipotle with rice, beans, chicken - everything delicious). What's interesting is that your diabetes devices are already giving you the answers to solve most of your problems with the data they collect. The only thing missing is your attention to the blood sugar ("retrospective analysis" will fix that) and the ability to interpret the data that has been shown to you (this book and/or coaching will help you to learn how to do that). So if we can look at our CGM graphs and identify not only the problem areas but also interpret them for the proper solutions, we're able to retrospectively analyze this information on a day-to-day or week-to-week basis and make adjustments to our diabetes management that actually work, and then we don't have to wait for our doctors to fix it for us (or fail to fix it because they lack the proper context).

*****

The Importance of Timing and Volume

In assessing your blood sugars with "**retrospective analysis**," you're looking for the problems that you can solve by either altering the *timing* or *volume* of the variables at play. That's it. Take insulin earlier or later. Take more or less insulin overall. Same thing with sugar or anything else that makes blood sugar rise and fall—*timing* and *volume*. Earlier or later, more or less. How cool (and simple) is that?

Real-life example continued: In analyzing my post-breakfast spikes, I can tell you that it spiked but came down relatively quickly. Here's the assessment: I spiked because I cut my pre-bolus timing in half that day so that I *would* spike by manipulating blood sugar (I'll share more in the next chapter on how you can manipulate blood sugar intentionally). I came down pretty fast because I was running around town carrying Brooklyn, my two-year-old daughter, and running errands. Activity like this does two big things: it burns glucose (lowering blood sugar), and it helps insulin to circulate and work faster (also lowering blood sugar). *This* is why my spike was intentional; I wanted to avoid a low blood sugar that would have happened if I had stayed perfectly stable at the initial 87 mg/dL from the earlier example, but these are things that my endo would never know. However, the pattern of morning spikes that I noticed over the previous two weeks means that I'm not taking enough insulin or I'm not giving the insulin enough time to work (your situation may be different). By assessing this information, I'm able to check off the first letter in the ARM framework.

This step of managing blood sugars is the "A" of the ARM framework, which I mentioned earlier stands for "Assess." We are assessing our CGM graphs and trying to identify both successes and potential problem areas that we've encountered throughout our days. We can learn from our mistakes, and they can be used productively to ensure a better tomorrow. All blood sugar, as mentioned before, exists for a reason. It doesn't just magically go terribly wrong; there's always a reason it goes up and down. It's our job now to identify the reason, whether it be a meal, insulin, exercise, or some combination of other variables as well. This first step can also be referred to as "getting curious" about your blood sugar as you begin to take more responsibility outside of the doctor's office. Become more aware and pay attention to your blood sugars because the numbers we experience are like a breadcrumb trail full of hints trying to tell you how to fix them.

Ultimately, this first step of "retrospective analysis" allows us to see and review problems that arise that we might have overlooked during the event (because life is crazy enough without stopping to analyze blood sugar every five minutes), and it allows us to identify which variable might be at the root cause of blood sugar that isn't cooperating. For example, if I take my insulin for lunch at noon and watch what happens when I eat the meal, I can use the timing of any spikes or drops that follow as an indicator of what I need to change to improve my outcomes. Let's explore the three "time windows" of mealtime "retrospective analysis":

Window #1: If I see a spike or a drop within one hour of taking my insulin, the first thing I look at is inappropriate pre-bolus *timing*. If my pre-bolus is too short, I might see a spike in that first hour because I didn't give my insulin enough time to do its work for the food I ate. Alternatively, if my pre-bolus is too long (I waited too long to eat my food), I might see a drop in blood sugar during that first hour because the insulin got a chance to work before the food started to digest. If you've ever dosed for a meal and forgotten to eat (or been distracted), you've probably also experienced that type of low, not fun.

Note: Pre-bolus timing is often recommended at 10 to 15 minutes, *no matter what*, and this is *wrong* and can be dangerous. Your pre-bolus timing *needs* to be dynamic depending on current blood sugar, insulin on board, activity level, type of food, and so much more, and may look a little different than the standard "10-15 minutes" (hint: mine is currently 20 minutes).

Window #2 of "retrospective analysis" timing that I want to look at is between one and two hours after I've taken that mealtime bolus. So, if I were to take my insulin at noon and eat my lunch, but I see a spike or a drop between hours one and two (1 and 2 p.m. in this example), it likely has to do with my insulin-to-carb ratio (the *volume* of insulin given). If I go high, there is likely not enough insulin present to take care of the foods I eat, but if I go low in that time frame, there is likely too much insulin present. Remember that these are generic rules of thumb; you are becoming your own doctor, and there are many other factors at play that we'll cover later in this book.

Window #3: We want to look at the time between hours two and three (in this example, from 2 p.m. to 3 p.m.), where we might consider the total dose for proteins and fats as the root cause, which is also where my endo got her initial assessment wrong many years ago and told me to take more long-acting insulin instead of a second dose of mealtime insulin for protein. To be fair, she didn't know the cause, as our medical teams are not always up to date on cutting-edge information like this. This time-frame study can give us good insight into our digestion rate as well. If you constantly see delayed spikes many hours later, with lows up front, you may want to ask your doctor about gastroparesis.

Now, the final time window here, anything beyond three hours, is likely going to be a mixture of higher fat diets or long-acting or basal insulin adjustments that are needed. What we want to consider is the spike or drop in our blood sugars *in relation to* the most recent dose of insulin and meal consumption. If the first hour is the issue, it might mean an adjustment to the pre-bolus as a potential solution (timing). If the problem area occurs in the second-hour time slot, it might require an adjustment to the insulin-to-carb ratio (volume). In the third hour, you might consider any highs as a miscalculation of insulin to proteins and fats. Last of all, seeing problems in the fourth hour and beyond means it's likely higher fat or the long-acting or basal insulin that would require adjustment. Remember also that our notes

ONLY apply to that exact meal consumed for that test. Different food types, time of day, recent exercise, etc., can also impact our data.

Obviously, these are not perfect timelines as there are many factors and variables that impact blood sugar, such as exercise, hydration, sleep, stress levels, insulin resistance, and so forth. However, this framework within "retrospective analysis" gave me a starting point in identifying what *might* be adjusted first while on my quest toward more stable blood sugar after meals in the absence of advanced help from my medical team. *And since I am not a doctor*, I can't tell you exactly how much insulin to take or when, but the framework allows you to start looking at your own blood sugar levels along with what is likely the root cause of them going out of range after a full meal. So again, allow me to reiterate that I am *not* a doctor, and *this is not medical advice*. My intention is to give you the information you need to act as your own medical practitioner and take more responsibility and control over your diabetes management (since no one is coming to save us, we must act on our own as "**Renegade Warriors**").

In chapter 6, I want to give you one of the greatest gifts I discovered on my journey toward more predictable diabetes management: how to manipulate blood sugars to do what *you* want them to do.

Notes:

_____

_____

_____

_____

_____

_____

_____

_____

_____

_____

_____

_____

_____

_____

_____

_____

_____

CHAPTER 6

BALANCING AND MANIPULATING BLOOD SUGARS

O n my way to the gym for what seemed like a standard workout, I noticed my blood sugar was sitting a lot higher than I typically aim for. I pulled into the gym parking lot feeling a bit nauseous, and saw that my blood sugar was stuck at 220. I ran a quick calculation in my head using my correction factor (also known as the insulin sensitivity factor), deciding how much insulin I needed to take to bring it back into a healthy spot before walking inside to start my warm-up. At this point in my life, I was training to be a firefighter and needed to improve my cardio, so I hopped on the treadmill to start things off. As I was doing a practice run for my firefighter's physical test, I got about ten minutes in before I started to feel really light on my feet. I felt like I could run forever. I assumed I was coming back into a healthy blood sugar range again as the nausea from my high blood sugar had also gone away.

Five minutes later, things felt very different. I realized that the superhuman feeling I was experiencing was actually my blood sugar plummeting. The light-on-my-feet athletic performance turned into a sinking feeling in my stomach as I lost sensation in my extremities, and the world started to get a little blurry. My body began to shake, and my skin was covered in sweat. I pulled out my CGM and saw that my blood sugar was no longer at 220 mg/dL but was plummeting toward an urgent low. I hopped off the treadmill just in time to test my blood sugar on the floor in the corner of the gym and saw that it had already dropped 130 points to 90 mg/dL. While 90 might seem like a healthy number to most, in the *context* of the situation, knowing that I took insulin and was exercising, it proved to be a dangerous combination with double arrows down showing on my CGM. For the first time ever, I learned about the accelerating force that exercise can have on insulin when recently dosed.

*****

Balancing Arrows

One of the most popular frameworks I'm known for in our type 1 diabetes community is the concept of "balancing arrows," which I'd like to introduce to you today. See, what happened leading up to the gym treadmill incident made sense in my head; I would take insulin for high blood sugar and continue on with my day. But what I didn't know yet was that when different variables combine with each other, the effects they have on our blood sugar can often change (for good or for bad). So, when I go for a run in an attempt to lower my blood sugar in the absence of additional fast-acting insulin, I do see an impact (a lowering impact). However, the amount dropped when I went for a run in the presence of extra insulin on board (like in this example where I gave a correction dose of insulin *and then* went for a run); the impact on blood sugar seemed to be compounded and accelerated. It's almost like the formula changes when two or more blood sugar variables are present at the same time.

Before this gets too complicated—and in an effort to simplify the entire concept—I'll give you an example. If I take insulin for my breakfast and time it correctly, then hypothetically, the two variables (insulin + food) should balance out nicely because insulin would drop my blood sugar, and breakfast would spike my blood sugar. So the two—an arrow down (insulin) and an arrow up (food)—would balance everything out to be stable and in range.

Now, let's take a look at the same example with the added variable of exercise immediately after eating that breakfast. Exercise (for me) typically lowers blood sugar. What I've found is that if I have more variables that lower blood sugar (insulin and exercise in this case), that are combined with variables that spike blood sugar (the carbs from breakfast in this example), then the overall result will be a lower blood sugar (two on the lowering side, one on the raising side, and therefore the lowering effect wins due to an imbalance in the equation).

So, when I introduced insulin to manage my high blood sugar, it should have been enough to address the elevated levels I was experiencing before going to the gym. However, when I added another variable that also lowers blood sugar, like running on the treadmill, I found myself in a precarious situation with my blood sugar plummeting to a dangerous level because I had *two* lowering factors working together. Had I known about this dangerous combination previously, I could have reduced (or removed) the correction dose if I anticipated the drop in blood sugar from the run. Alternatively, if I was unaware of these impacts, but actively watching my numbers, I could have proactively "balanced" out that drop a little earlier on the treadmill with some sugar.

The goal is to "balance the equation." If I've got blood sugars heading down, I need to identify and implement a new variable that will cause my blood sugars to go up in an equal amount. This single arrow down variable would hypothetically be balanced out (or canceled out) by the single arrow up variable, resulting in a stable blood sugar number overall. This is ideally what happens when we eat food. We take insulin (an arrow down variable) and eat food (an arrow up variable), and (*ideally*) blood sugar is stable without big drops or spikes (assuming we time them correctly with the pre-bolus). The fun part, though, is that this method can be used for *all* blood sugar situations, not just at mealtime. In fact, the idea behind "balancing arrows" is that as we experience undesirable blood sugar in everyday life, we identify variables (via retrospective analysis that you just learned about in the last few chapters) and implement strategies to balance them out. *This* (in a nutshell) is how my clients get their first in-range wins when working with us. It is, quite frankly, the fastest path to 90% time in range (defined by the ADA to be between 70—180 mg/dL) without my clients having to learn "everything." In all truth, you only need a basic knowledge of a few up variables and a few down variables to start seeing results *right now*. So, let's break down a few of my favorites (this is a generic list from *my* experience and may differ for you).

UP blood sugar variables:
- Carbohydrates (simple and complex carbohydrates)
- Stress (physical, mental, social, and so on)
- Adrenaline
- Resistance/HIIT (anaerobic) exercise

DOWN blood sugar variables:
- Cardiovascular (aerobic) exercise
- Insulin
- Hydration (in the presence of adequate insulin)
- Certain medications

Now, here's where it gets a little tricky…

Not all ups and downs are going to cause blood sugar to rise or fall at the same speed.

It might take insulin 15 to 90 minutes to really do some damage and bring a high blood sugar reading down into range, whereas (for me), going for a quick run can drop me 50+ blood sugar points in about ten minutes flat.

GOLDEN NUGGET: The *timing* of the impact on blood sugar and the *volume* of the impact is going to differ between all variables.

On the other hand, some ups (like juice, glucose, or other fast-acting carbs) might cause a rapid rise, while others (like proteins) might lead to a very slow and delayed rise.

Big picture: the first piece of this that I want to convey to anybody trying to learn about the "**balancing arrows**" framework is that we are looking for an *equal and opposite* directional arrow with our blood sugar equation. So if I have something that causes a rapid spike, like a simple and fast carbohydrate like a fruit smoothie, then I need to find an *equal and opposite* reaction to cause a rapid decline or drop in blood sugar if I want to balance it out. This can be done with more than one strategy. For example, I could pair insulin + going for a walk to make insulin work faster if I've already consumed my smoothie, or I could take insulin earlier to give it more of a head start so that it's already lowering blood sugar before I start to enjoy my smoothie. Different situations call for different strategies.

Here's a great example that happened to me recently. If you're familiar with time in range, I wanted to challenge myself and decided to go for 100% time in range for seven consecutive days. This means that I wanted to stay between 70 and 180 mg/dL 24 hours a day through all of my meals, Ironman workouts, and day-to-day life. By days six and seven, I was a little stressed with all of the pressure of being so close to my goal. I didn't want to lose it, so I relied *heavily* on the "balancing arrows" framework. I had running shoes on one side of my desk and a bowl of candy on the other because if my blood sugar began to creep up and go toward the higher ranges, I'd grab my running shoes, run out the door, and run around the block because I knew that if I went for a short run, my blood sugar would drop almost immediately.

Using this simple trick on that day brought a spiking blood sugar that was sure to go out of range back down, not only to a level number but all the way to a healthy range within 15 minutes. Alternatively, if my blood sugar was dropping rapidly, I had the bowl of candy next to me as an option to rapidly bring my blood sugar back up. While this isn't a long-term solution (because who wants to babysit blood sugar every day forever), it's a great way to calm chaotic blood sugars in a pinch (like hitting the reset button for blood sugars).

*****

Looking for More Options

Where I see a lot of people get lost is in thinking that the only options we have to control blood sugar are insulin and sugar. Thinking that those are the only two "balancing arrows" in our diabetes toolbox. The truth is that although they may be some of the most effective, we have a lot of different options to choose from and should vary our approaches to match the urgency of the rise or fall. If I'm slowly falling below 100 mg/dL, I might not need a full juice box or tube full of glucose tabs to bring me up. Maybe a single bite of fruit will do the trick. If I'm spiking past 200, but I have insulin on board, maybe a quick walk around the neighborhood will bring me back down to a healthy level (because activity often helps insulin to work faster), and I won't need to stack insulin aggressively.

> **REMEMBER: As "renegade warriors,"**
> **we think differently.**

And when we combine different options and variables, it can actually make the blood sugar reactions stronger (whether we intend to, or not). Remember when I told you about my experience with insulin and running? I now know that that combo typically produces a scary, fast drop; I dropped

130 points in less than 30 minutes and likely would have continued well into an urgent low had I not immediately grabbed a juice box from my gym bag. When we consider the *equal and opposite* reaction and what's needed to balance things out in a situation like that, I might drink juice, consume glucose tabs, or have a cookie. What you might be thinking at this point, though, and what's interesting to me, is that we have a lot more options for pushing blood sugar up than we do for pushing it down.

Insulin is the primary option for precision control. Dial in your exact insulin ratios, formulas, and calculations, and you'll master diabetes in no time because, hypothetically, you'll know exactly how much to add or reduce in order to balance things out in any situation (like a normal functioning pancreas would do). That's the missing piece that categorizes us as "type 1 diabetic." The issue is that this is incredibly difficult to do because there are *so* many other factors to consider outside of just insulin that impact blood sugar, as well as how much insulin we actually need at any given moment (due to shifts in insulin resistance/insulin sensitivity that we'll cover in the next chapter).

Exercise is a good secondary option in this example for pushing blood sugar down, and in my experience, it's a great "rescue" method to get blood sugar back in range quickly, especially if only a small redirection is needed. And depending on the situation, it can sometimes be used *in place of additional insulin* to encourage blood sugar to go down. Not forever, because unfortunately, there's no cure through exercise, but it can be a temporary solution to improve insulin sensitivity and burn glucose.

After learning this, I had a few instances where I opted to eat a meal while riding my bike and let the exercise keep my blood sugar in check instead of taking additional mealtime insulin. The context here is that my idea of a "bike ride" has changed dramatically since training for my Ironman races began, and can linger on for 4, 5, 6+ hours on the bike - which is no wonder why I can eat food and not have to dose extra for it while covering 60, 80, 100+ miles of exercise. An important note to add, however, is that I do still have basal insulin going through my insulin pump at those times; there's just no additional bolus (mealtime) insulin.

That being said, when we look at this through the lens of the "**balancing arrows**" concept, diabetes becomes a game of manipulating blood sugar in real-time. When we understand that all we have to do is introduce an *equal and opposite* **reaction**, it's no longer about wondering how I get my blood sugar back in range but more of a question of what I need to do to balance out the current blood sugar trajectory. And in some cases, as wild as it sounds, it's not about what I need to do but about what I need to make sure I *don't* do. In other words, if my blood sugar is currently spiking, and I'm about to eat dinner, I probably shouldn't start eating my food before I take my insulin because that's going to make matters worse.

Alternatively, if I'm currently going low with insulin on board, maybe I don't start with doing the dishes and cleaning up after dinner (movement might make the low come on faster and more significantly) but instead relax and have a slow conversation while I fix the low. So, we look at diabetes as one giant chart of up and down arrows that we get to pick from to balance out any situation in which we find ourselves. We're able to see which variables need to be present if we're trying to stabilize blood sugar and which ones we need to delay or remove to keep a stable line going steady.

It gets tricky in the second phase of understanding the "**balancing arrows**" framework because not all variables are as easy to understand as simply up or down. Some variables might be double arrows up, meaning a rapid rise, while other variables might be double arrows down, which is a rapid drop. If I have a run workout for my upcoming race event, I expect to counterbalance that (anticipated) double arrows down with something that's double arrows up. I have a special mixed solution in my water that's straight sugar (dextrose plus electrolytes), and I consume it one sip at a time throughout my run to balance the arrows and keep me (nearly) perfectly in range. Short "bursts" of a rapid rise variable (dextrose drink) to balance out the constant pushing down variable (running).

BALANCING ARROW (CGM)	RATE OF CHANGE (PER 5 MINUTES)	VISUALS
→	+/- 0-4 mg/dL	
↗	+ 5-9 mg/dL	
↘	− 5-9 mg/dL	
↑	+ 10-14 mg/dL	
↓	− 10-14 mg/dL	
↑↑	+ 15 mg/dL (OR MORE)	
↓↓	− 15 mg/dL (OR MORE)	

CONVERSION FOR m/moL: DIVIDE mg/dL by 18

(Rates of change based on and courtesy of Dexcom)

In addition to the rapid rise and fall arrows, we also have blood sugar variables that bring about arrows that are only slanted up and slanted down, representing a slow increase and decrease in blood sugar, respectively. A common example of this might be taking the trash out or walking around the block with the family, which might lead to a slow and steady drop (as it does for me). Traditionally, if you wanted to go for a walk and not experience a low blood sugar, the medical advice would be to have a "snack" that's high in protein.

There are two issues with this advice, the first being that the term "snack" is generic—there's no precise amount of food that they're recommending (which is good because the amount needed will change depending on the person and type/duration of the activity itself).

Second, for decades, diabetics have been told that proteins are the food that stabilizes blood sugar. But this couldn't be further from the truth. The reason that it seems like it stabilizes blood sugar is that through a process called gluconeogenesis, protein converts to glucose—eventually. Proteins don't "stabilize" blood sugar; they lead to a slow and delayed rise (or a delayed slanted arrow UP). The problem is that it can take hours to see the impact, so it goes largely unnoticed in our blood sugar if we don't know what to look for in our CGM reports. So many doctors, endocrinologists, dietitians, and other medical professionals miss this. As I mentioned earlier in the book, my endo didn't even think about protein when I was experiencing these "drifting" high blood sugars hours after meals. Instead, she ended up increasing my long-acting insulin, thinking my higher blood sugar was just a basal rate problem (since it was so far removed from mealtime). Thus, when protein does lead to an eventual rise in blood sugar, we don't always see it right away as the true causation and often mislabel it with something incorrect.

The "balancing effect" that's attributed to proteins and blood sugar is often a rise from the protein that's offsetting what would otherwise have been a slow drop from activity. So, if I go for a walk, but before the walk, I had a high-protein snack, there's a good chance that the protein, via a slow conversion to glucose, might offset (or cancel out, balance, etc.) the slow drop I would have experienced from the walk. Alternatively, if I consumed that same high-protein snack in the absence of a walk, I might notice an hour or two later that it would actually raise my blood sugar (because there would be no walk to balance it out with a slow drop). The walk by itself would lower my blood sugar a little bit, and the protein by itself would raise my blood sugar a little bit, but in timing those together, they would hypothetically stabilize (or cancel out), which is why proteins are assumed to stabilize blood sugar. The reality is that we've just been balancing the arrows this whole time and didn't even know it.

Let's organize those thoughts below:

- A walk by itself = drop in blood sugar
- Eating a high-protein snack by itself = a rise in blood sugar
- Eat a high-protein snack *and then* go for a walk = stable blood sugar

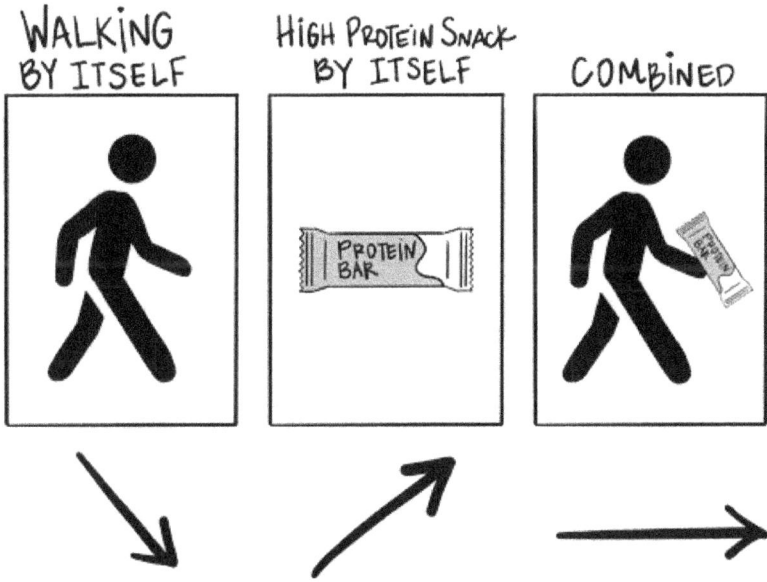

*****

Cancel Out the Bad With the Good

My goal with diabetes (and likely yours as well) becomes a balancing act in the big picture as well when we think of "stable blood sugars *plus* flexibility and freedom in life." In the more detailed (smaller) picture, I want to figure out how to cancel out any errors or undesirable blood sugars as they arise. The caveat here is that up or down arrows in different situations might be considered good or bad, and the label of good or bad changes with the context of each situation. As an example, if I have double arrows down, which is a rapid drop in blood sugar, and my current blood sugar is 200 mg/dL, this would be good news because I would likely be in a situation where I wanted blood sugars to come down and get back into a healthy range. *Context* is critical. Alternatively, if I had an enormous amount of insulin on board from a recent bolus and I was double arrows down (rapid drop) at 70 mg/dL, I'd probably consider that to be a little scarier of a situation. All in all, it's not that these blood sugar variables are inherently good or bad but that they exist as options in our tool chest to use to balance out undesirable blood sugar fluctuations.

Let's look at another example as an equation. If we have up arrows on the left side of an equation and down arrows on the right side of the equation, I'm able to zero out (balance) the equation. Said differently: I'm trying to cancel out the variables so my blood sugar stays stable—where I want it. In math terms, if I have a +1 and a -1, they cancel out to equal 0. This is the goal of diabetes, where zero represents "stable" because there's "zero" change in blood sugars (hypothetically). The only time we don't want to balance the equation is if you're currently at a blood sugar level you don't like. In this case, you might want to introduce more of the opposite variable to push blood sugar toward a desirable range. If I'm currently at 75 mg/dL and about to go for a run, I'd like to "push" blood sugars up over 130 mg/dL to where I feel more confident with a little added buffer for a drop in blood sugar, should it occur. I don't want to balance my arrows to stay at 75 mg/dL; I want to push blood sugars in one direction (technically, this means it would be an unbalanced equation since I *want* an up arrow only) until I am satisfied with where the blood sugar lands.

Another example would be if I'm at 65 mg/dL with low blood sugar before dinner; I don't want to "balance my arrows" and stay steady at 65. If I'm about to eat food and I know my perfect insulin-to-carb ratio, then the food and the insulin would balance out if I gave the proper amount of insulin. But I don't want them to balance and keep me at low blood sugar levels, right? So, in this example, I might offset the balance and consider taking less insulin so that I end up at a slightly higher blood sugar two hours later (as a result of the partially missing insulin, my blood sugar would have a higher endpoint 2 hours later. The question that remains, of course, is how much to reduce the insulin so as not to skyrocket and end up hyperglycemic). The ultimate goal is to manipulate blood sugar to achieve the desired outcome that *you* want. With this framework, we have the power to decide what happens to our blood sugar. And because every blood sugar number exists for a reason, it becomes our responsibility to identify *why* it moves up or down, as well as what we can do about it with the **"balancing arrows" framework**.

The tricky part about diabetes is that we don't know all of the variables and "balancing arrows" on day one when we're diagnosed. Heck, I've spoken with people 50+ years into their diagnosis who have still never been taught any of these concepts or strategies (nothing against them; it's their medical team that failed them). This is where having a coach can come in handy, as well as taking excellent notes of what you see in your blood sugar management for discussion with your coach (because they should be able to identify and interpret the blood sugar numbers you give them).

Experimentation comes into play as well. And since this book is *not* medical advice, but based on my experience as a type 1 diabetic and from my experience coaching other type 1 diabetics, I can tell you that I experimented daily for years to map out exactly what variables cause blood sugar to go up or down or stay stable (meal after meal, day after day, month after month, yes - YEARS). As you document these practices while you read through this book, you will slowly begin to map out what works for you and the options you have available to remedy any undesirable blood sugar levels that may arise.

As you start to learn about these new factors, I want you to understand that blood sugars don't go out of range for no reason. Everything has a root cause. The reason might be unknown to you at this time, but as you learn from this book and learn from the resources granted to you inside (and outside) this book, we are able to assign more meaning to the fluctuations we encounter. If you remember, at the beginning of this book, I talked about "**diabetes math**." We can imagine the up arrow as "plus one" and the down arrow as "minus one." In this example, with "diabetes math," the goal is to reach zero. Addition and subtraction—or using "balancing arrows"— whichever is easier for you to understand and implement in your own life, is the basis of "diabetes math" and blood sugar formulas. It's how we can begin to redirect and manipulate our blood sugar at will to accomplish more stable and predictable blood sugar that remains in range for longer periods of time. *This* is how we get our life back.

My job is to take complicated "diabetes math" and simplify it to a level of easy understanding and implementation, but the reality is that diabetes is crazy complicated, and it took me over a decade to condense this information and these strategies into easy-to-implement pieces. When we think about the fact that there are more than 50 blood sugar variables, and each has its own set of up-and-down arrows and interactions, it can get confusing and overwhelming. Right now, I want you to zoom out and think about the different pieces and experiences in your life where you have seen the impact of "balancing arrows." I'll give you your first one: you probably take insulin (down arrow) so that you can eat carbs (up arrow) like me. Now, dig deeper for other examples; they're everywhere. The more you can identify, the easier diabetes management gets. Happy hunting.

In the next chapter, I'll show you what's likely led to those "mysterious" blood sugar fluctuations that seem to have no rhyme or reason, and how you can demystify diabetes for good.

Notes:

_____

_____

_____

_____

_____

_____

_____

_____

_____

_____

_____

_____

_____

_____

_____

_____

_____

CHAPTER 7

THREE LEVELS OF IMPACT

While writing this book, my life in the last year and a half has been dedicated to training for and competing in triathlons with an upcoming Ironman (my first one ever). These are races that I never thought I would ever consider because I was never an endurance athlete growing up. But during this training process, my body went through some major transformations. Initially, because I was doing so much running, biking, and swimming, my blood sugar would drop all over the place, seemingly without warning. In the first week or two of my training, I had blood sugar that would get stuck low and not come up for hours on end, to the point where I was consuming 50 grams of carbohydrates just to keep it from going lower (a good indication that insulin needs to be adjusted, in my experience). What makes sense now, and what's interesting when looking back, is that after a couple of weeks, I had also gained eight pounds, not muscle, but fat.

For the first time in my life, I was concerned about weight gain, and I needed to figure out my strategies to get things more dialed in. I knew that consuming enormous amounts of sugar just to fix my drops and lows wasn't going to be the solution for me (this is called "feeding the insulin," where you're required to eat carbs throughout the day just to avoid lows, which leads to excess calories that can make weight management a difficult battle). Even more interesting is that the low blood sugar didn't happen only when I was exercising. Sometimes, it would happen hours or even days later.

This is a lesson that stood out to me as I was building my blood sugar plans for the actual races themselves, as they can go on for multiple hours (my next race is expected to be between 12 and 18 hours long). You see, blood sugar is more than what we see day to day in the moment. Sometimes there are things impacting it that are a result of bigger picture variables from hours ago or even days ago. So, when I had increased my exercise on a more consistent basis, what I had actually done in the background (and we'll cover this more in this chapter) was increase my insulin sensitivity at a base level.

Ultimately, during exercise, I'm burning glucose (energy) for my activity. After exercise, my body is primed in a more "insulin sensitive" state where I need less insulin for the same amounts of food I might have had the day before. In an "insulin sensitive" state, I consider slightly altering my insulin-to-carb ratio, basal rates, and correction factor (depending on the total impact). I did end up having to make an adjustment in this situation, but what I want you to take away from this is that our insulin sensitivity (and, on the opposite side of the spectrum, our insulin resistance) can change day to day, but it can also be manipulated intentionally (and to your benefit) if you use what I'm about to show you.

When I mention the "spectrum" between insulin sensitivity and insulin resistance, I see many doctors and medical professionals leading with the fact that you either are or are not insulin resistant. And the issue isn't in identifying if we are or are not, but rather looking at it on a spectrum of *how much* or *how little* we are insulin resistant or insulin sensitive. And if we imagine it on a scale of more resistant to insulin or more sensitive to insulin, we actually see that as we become less insulin resistant, we are, therefore, more insulin sensitive as a result. On the opposite side, as we become less insulin sensitive, we become more insulin resistant. So, it's more of a question of whether we're moving toward insulin resistance or toward insulin sensitivity with each of our blood sugar variables and daily decisions like exercise, sleep, stress level, and on and on.

This is known as the first of the three levels of impact: past behaviors that affect our current level of insulin resistance or insulin sensitivity. For example, changes in my usual routine, such as intense workouts while training for triathlons, can dramatically impact present blood sugar levels. If this is confusing, I've got a few examples coming up that should provide some clarity. Take a moment to really take this all in; this could be the chapter that changes your life forever.

*****

Past, Present, and Predictability

What I want you to understand is that our lifestyle habits and choices can impact our blood sugar for hours or sometimes days on end. I may not have slept well for a couple of days in a row—maybe because of travel or work, or in my case, a toddler—and this might impact how my blood sugar responds the following day (lack of adequate sleep leads to higher insulin resistance). This is the resulting blood sugar that might go unnoticed if you don't recognize the impact that lack of sleep can have. The reason sleep specifically impacts blood sugar, because I know it sounds silly the first time you hear it, is that a lack of sleep increases cortisol production, and an increase of cortisol increases our insulin resistance, which in turn makes our insulin needs higher, which means if we make no adjustment (because we might be ignorant to the impact in the first place), our blood sugar will also be higher that following day for what seems like "no reason at all." So, in this chain of events, we can see that one *past* habit or event impacted our insulin resistance, which then impacted our *present* blood sugar. This is just one example of level one in the three levels of impact.

Another example would be how (when I started training for triathlons) my workouts increased my insulin sensitivity and produced lows for days and even weeks on end. *Past* (level one blood sugar impact—my increase in exercise) impacting the *present* (level two blood sugar impact, but we'll get to that in a second) blood sugar. When we know how our *past* decisions and habits impact our *present* blood sugar, we can set up our daily habits to benefit our everyday lives with blood sugar management by looking for habits that improve insulin sensitivity and, therefore, reduce insulin resistance. Your head might be spinning after reading that, and to be honest, mine did as well when I first had this "ah-ha" moment, but I promise to simplify it all (I even have some fancy illustrations for you). What's interesting is that the concepts that I'm about to lay out are the most common reasons I see clients of mine experiencing "unexplained" highs and lows that led to absolute frustration before working with me. But this only works if we can use this knowledge to impact blood sugar *intentionally*. When I didn't expect blood sugar to be impacted so heavily by my workouts, the lows caught me by surprise. Knowing what to expect means that we now have more opportunities to control or manipulate blood sugar, and opens up opportunities to do so with something other than "only" insulin. If I want to take less insulin today, I could even pick habits and actions that will improve my insulin sensitivity enough to *balance* my blood sugars (to a certain degree, of course—still take what you need in terms of insulin) in place of only taking additional insulin.

Do you see how exciting this is? It's literally a balancing game, and by the end of this chapter, you'll see how using the three levels of blood sugar impact will enable you to *force* blood sugars to do what you want, even when it gets stubborn. And with the level one blood sugar impacts noted as a scale or "slider" (as you'll see in the following image), it gives us an opportunity to visually set ourselves up for success before we even start to take insulin or count carbs or do anything for our diabetes each day.

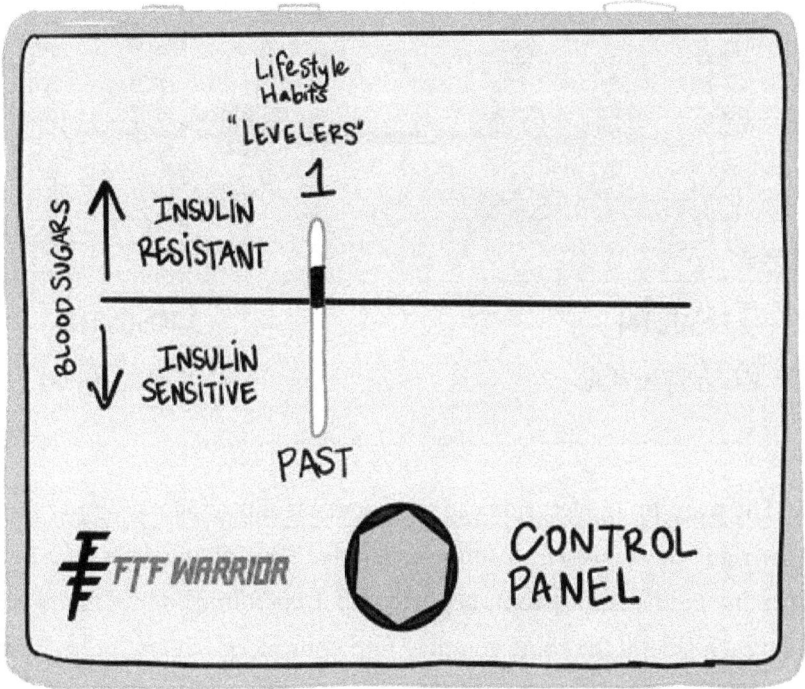

Are you noticing a little higher blood sugar on average (like your fasting blood sugar first thing in the morning)? Maybe consider any new habits in life that could have led to increased insulin resistance (like higher fat content in your diet, less activity, more stress, or less sleep). What can you do? *Equal and opposite reactions in the level one spectrum.* Do something that will either *reduce* insulin resistance (get more sleep) or something that will *increase* insulin sensitivity (like increase exercise). Level one can be summarized as **"lifestyle variables."** Alternatively, yes, you can also consider more insulin for the highs if that fits your strategy better.

An example that I gave during a recent training with my private clients is that our level one "lifestyle variables" can be imagined as a group of friends playing tug-o-war with each other.

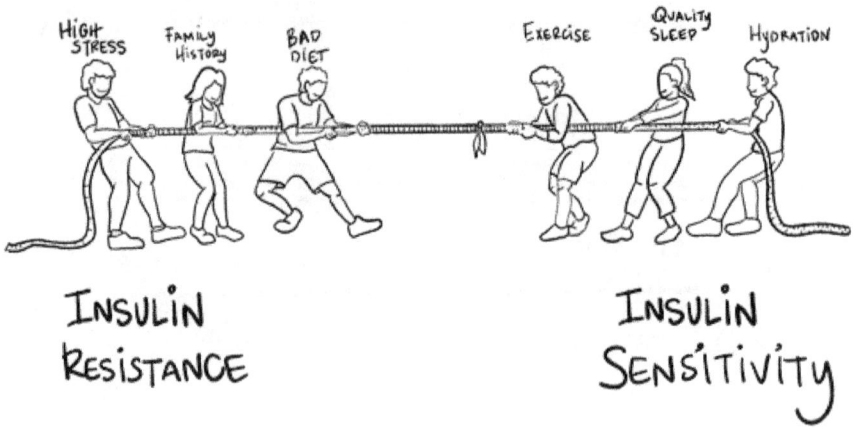

The team on the left side can represent insulin resistance, and the team on the right can represent insulin sensitivity. Your blood sugars are smack-dab in the middle as the people begin to pull. Depending on how many people are on each side of the rope, you may find your blood sugars "pulled" to one side or the other (either more insulin resistant, or more insulin sensitive) on any given day. The amount of friends on each team is a representation of your current lifestyle variables that day/week. You might wake up one morning after a terrible night of sleep, sick and stressed out, and on the back end of binge-eating BBQ for dinner the night before and find that you're much closer to the insulin resistance side.

In that example, you're "insulin resistance" tug-o-war team is looking pretty strong, and will likely "win," so you'll need to prepare some strategies to even the playing field for the "insulin sensitivity" team (or suffer the consequences of higher blood sugars due to the teams being out of balance). The secret is that at any given time, we can also manipulate the variables by adjusting the insulin that we give (or don't give) as a last resort (though it is more difficult to change insulin dosing "on the fly" with accuracy and without a perfect blood sugar formula in place already).

*****

Choosing Healthy Habits

Simply by incorporating more healthy lifestyle habits into our lives, we give ourselves a better chance of seeing lower fasting blood glucose levels, lower postprandial spikes (postprandial refers to "after meal" blood sugar spikes), and a variety of other benefits in our overall body functionality. What's interesting is that these same habits work just as well for non-diabetics as they do for diabetics. So, whether you take insulin manually or your pancreas produces it, you can give this lesson to your friends and family as an encouragement to follow along in this book with you and support you in your health endeavors as they support their own health alongside you. If we can set up lifestyle habits that set up our blood sugar for success, we will also (as a by-product) improve the optimal functionality of our bodily systems as a whole and set ourselves up for an easier life in the long run—hard choices made in the now equal an easier life later on.

I'll give you an example from my own life right now that, to be honest, I'm struggling with—going to bed on time. I have a really difficult time saying no to using nighttime for hanging out with my wife and daughter, scrolling on social media, working, or watching TV. If I were to go to bed on time— which is a hard decision for me to make—I know that better sleep quality would impact tomorrow for the better. This is something that I either need to account for in my balancing equation (by increasing insulin to make up for inadequate sleep, exercise more, reduce fat intake, etc.) *or* just go to sleep earlier. So right now, for level one impacts, I want you to consider what habits in your life need improvement (or a complete change) that could ultimately be utilized to manage blood sugar better. In this level one blood sugar impact section, we call these our "levelers" because this will level the playing field for your blood sugar averages as you manipulate and improve insulin sensitivity at your base level. It allows us to set ourselves up for success through intentional planning ahead (which can be used to proactively plan to be more/less insulin sensitive for the next day) or by redirecting chaotic blood sugars by manipulating the "root cause" (an important thing to know when making adjustments to something as volatile as insulin dosing).

Let's end with one more example before getting into our level two blood sugar impacts. Since it does exist on a scale, if I know that I'm going to be insulin resistant because of my lifestyle choices, I need to balance out the equation by introducing more insulin sensitivity. For example, I had a client (we'll call him Jake) who attended a potluck barbecue where the foods were extremely high in fat and proteins. Because high-fat diets can lead to more insulin resistance, and high-protein diets lead to a delayed rise in blood sugar, we came up with a few different strategies depending on what Jake wanted to go with.

Knowing that it would lead to higher blood sugar (and higher levels of insulin resistance for the rest of the day), we took a look at the level two options to balance things out. We ended up calculating a temporary basal rate increase (only available to insulin pump users; for MDI, we would have calculated split bolus strategies) to take care of what would have been a stubborn delayed rise in blood sugar, but we could have just as easily increased insulin sensitivity the day before or the day of with an added workout that would have "balanced out" his insulin resistance (because the workout would increase insulin sensitivity, while the food choices would increase insulin resistance - when paired, they balance out). When I travel to the South and want to eat deep-fried, high-fat foods, I make sure to get a good workout each day to "cancel it out." Ultimately, I'm trying to "push" my insulin sensitivity back to the baseline (average) that I've got my insulin ratios and rates set to so that blood sugar *also* stays balanced without having to do a full reset on insulin-to-carb ratios, basal rates, correction factors, etc.

Yes, I can make adjustments to my insulin-to-carb ratios, basal rates, and correction factors, and I may even adjust my pre-bolus times. But to me, that's far more complicated than just balancing out my insulin resistance with some new insulin sensitivity so that I can keep all of my insulin (and blood sugar) simplified and steady.

Something to consider: Are you noticing blood sugar responds wildly differently from day to day under the same circumstances? Maybe you eat the same exact breakfast every single day, yet sometimes it spikes, and other times it's stable, and it's driving you nuts?

This used to drive me up the wall because it felt like there was never any predictability in my blood sugar. But after over a decade of research and experimentation, this concept of level one blood sugar impacts (the *past* impacts on our present blood sugar) finally brought me some clarity. It isn't that blood sugar is impossible to predict or control and changes day to day; it was that I was unknowingly causing my blood sugar to respond differently because my insulin resistance/sensitivity was changing day to day, and I didn't know how to anticipate it or respond to it so that it balanced out with the changing nature of life.

Here's an example from my life: the triathlon training made me more insulin sensitive, as mentioned above. So, I had a few choices. One was to eat more sugar, which I did, causing weight gain. I was experiencing low blood sugars for two weeks before adjusting my insulin to level things off and noticing the eight pounds I had put on. The weight gain led me to be more insulin resistant, and I had to adjust my insulin-to-carb ratios and my basal insulin pump settings once again to avoid the highs I started seeing as a result of putting on some weight. Then, I lost weight to show my clients in our T1D Weight Loss Challenge how to lose weight with type 1 diabetes, fast. This time, I was ready for the shift in insulin sensitivity that losing fat can bring, and had changed my insulin settings *while* I was losing weight so that I stayed balanced the entire time.

Special Note: A common pitfall that I see (and warned my clients of in our T1D weight loss challenge) is that as you finally start to see progress and lose weight, you must revisit your insulin needs and consider adjustments proactively. If you miss this window, the resulting "wacky" blood sugars could very well lead you to put the weight right back on. This is especially true if your insulin sensitivity increases and you begin "feeding the insulin" with extra, undesired calories to avoid the low blood sugars as I mentioned earlier.

Now, I mentioned level two blood sugar impacts earlier on, and I want to get to these because, honestly, they're even more exciting. Level two includes the choices we make in real-time to fix, redirect, and manipulate the direction that blood sugars are going in the *present* moment (you might remember this from the previous chapter). This is your "balancing arrows" framework in real-time. If I know I'm more insulin resistant because of a choice I made in the last few days (like junk food, less exercise, bad sleep, and so on), I can use my "balancing arrows" to encourage blood sugar to come back down with an *equal and opposite* reaction. This is especially helpful while you're still mapping out your level-one variables if you don't know what will make you more insulin resistant. You might wake up one day with a higher blood sugar and think, *Well darn, now what?* But it's really just a chance for you to practice your "balancing arrows" framework in the level two impact zone.

*****

Recovering From Mistakes

Here's where it gets exciting (see the following image for visual): we're able to redirect blood sugar in the *present* for mistakes or missed impacts in the *past*. Meaning that we can recover from just about any blood sugar blunder that we find ourselves in, even if it's rooted in something that happened earlier. If I forgot to take insulin for my lunch, I might take the insulin I need and go for a quick walk to get the insulin working faster. And if I don't sleep well for a couple of days and my insulin resistance increases, I know that for those couple of days, I might consider giving myself extra insulin, drinking extra water, or going for extra-long walks each day to improve my insulin sensitivity or balance my insulin needs. It's all about balancing the equation.

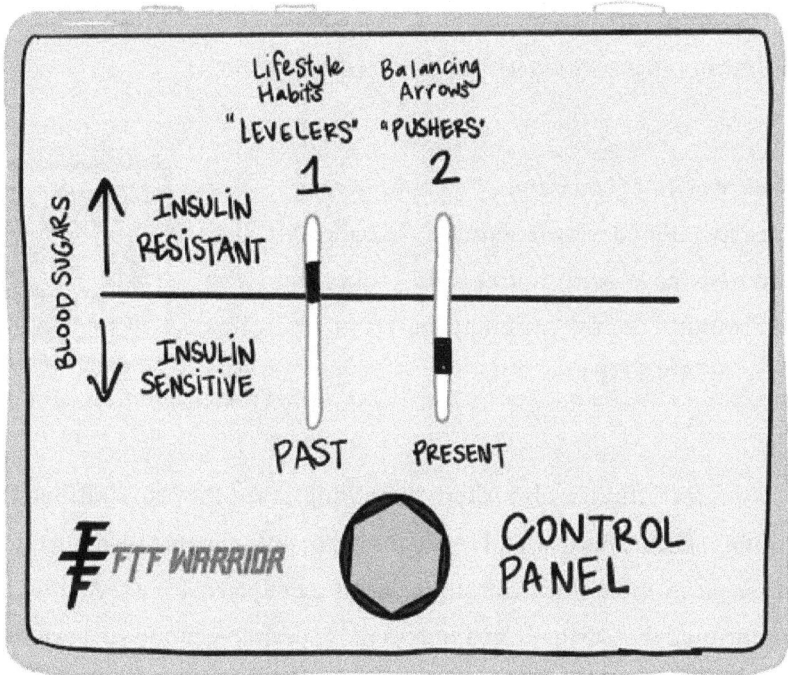

The image shows we have *equal and opposite* forces with level one and level two. This gives us a chance to predict more stable blood sugars in the future, which is what we'll get into in level three. So, as I consider level two variables (the "pushers" as we call them), I am "pushing" my blood sugars in the direction I want them to go in real time because of previous choices I had made in the *past* that have influenced my *present*. In the previous image above, you see that according to my level one variables, I'm experiencing some insulin resistance (maybe due to lack of sleep). I use level two variables to "balance" out the equation (maybe by introducing more insulin, exercise, or other blood sugar lowering variable) so that the resulting blood sugar is more stable. The final level, level three blood sugar impacts, is where our *predicted* blood sugars come into play. Ideally, using what we know from a "balancing arrows" framework (level two impact) and what we understand about our lifestyle habits impacting blood sugars (level one impact), we can *predict* more stable blood sugars as we anticipate the interactions of the different impacts.

Using the first two levels alone, you should be able to achieve at least a 90% time in range as soon as *tomorrow* if done correctly.

Unsure of how? I guarantee 90% time in range in our five-day "Blood Sugar Formula Challenge" that hundreds have paid to access. It's yours *free* since you're one of us now; my gift to you for grabbing this book. SCAN THE QR CODE:

Now, level three is also where something called the "**80/20 Blood Sugar Formula**" exists. This is what I set up for my private clients to get personalized blood sugar formulas for their unique goals set in place. It's a *predictive* blood sugar formula that virtually guarantees more desirable blood sugar outcomes through different activities (anything from walking the dog to a full Ironman race), foods (vegan, carnivore, flexible macros, any diet works), and experiences in life (aka - *living* life to the fullest). But for the purpose of this book, since I don't know you or what you're going through right now, I want you to focus on level one and level two, which we've just simplified as your *past* decisions and your *present* options.

Looking at the image, we can see that between levels one, two, and three, we have our *past*, our *present*, and our *predicted* blood sugars.

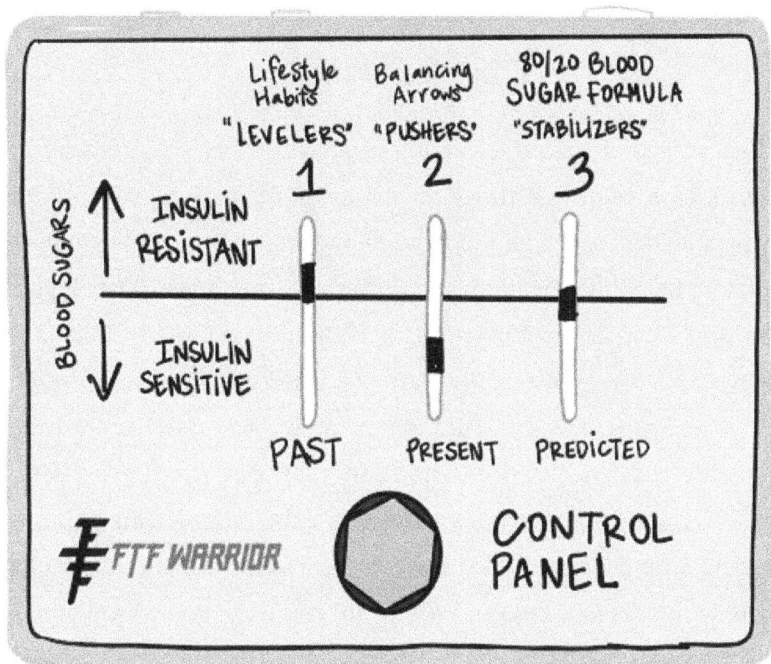

Level one impacts are the "levelers," the outside forces and previous decisions acting on my blood sugar and causing it to drift up or down throughout the day. Our "lifestyle variables" influence our baseline insulin resistance and insulin sensitivity.

Level two impacts are the "pushers" that enable us to actually *do* something about frustrating blood sugars and empower us to take control in a very real sense (of our diabetes, but also of our life and outcomes). These are the options we have to balance (or cancel) out what's happening as a residual impact from level one impacts. These are your "balancing arrows" in action.

And then level three, where we *predict* our blood sugar as we get into a deeper understanding in a more customized sense. This is where we discover our unique blood sugar formulas for a more automated, carefree, and flexible lifestyle while thriving with diabetes. Think of it like a blood sugar blueprint that *tells you* what to do in order to keep blood sugars so stable that you might occasionally forget that you have diabetes (in a good way).

In the absence of this knowledge of the three levels of blood sugar impact, however, we might see blood sugar go up or down unexpectedly, and we get mad, or at least I do. I get frustrated and anxious when I don't know why my blood sugar is doing what it's doing, especially when I'm uncertain what I should do to remedy the situation. An example that's all too common for many people I talk to is that they'll see blood sugar go up and up and up after a meal, and they'll give insulin, and it doesn't come down. They'll give more insulin, and when nothing happens, they'll give even more insulin. It can feel like they're injecting nothing but water because nothing seems to work.

The reality is that there are other factors—outside factors from level one—that act as hidden variables, and they can destroy us with these mysterious fluctuations because we don't see them immediately. If this leads to us solving for the wrong root cause, it can even land us in the hospital (like continuing to dose and dose and dose until you crash into a low blood sugar). What's helpful is to use your "retrospective analysis" that you learned earlier in this book to look backward at the last twelve hours, twenty-four hours, and beyond to see what other variables might be leading to the undesirable blood sugar so that you can actually fix it once and for all. *All blood sugars that we experience exist for a reason.* It's up to us to properly identify and remedy them.

I had a female client years ago who really enjoyed high-protein and high-fat meals that would cause her blood sugar to go up and get stuck for hours on end. She'd give a correction and see nothing happen, making her wonder if she needed to change her insulin vial or basal rates. She was truly uncertain about how to fix it. As you've probably caught on by now, it's not always that the insulin isn't working, but sometimes the extra insulin that's been given just keeps your blood sugar from getting worse. I had to remind her that when she hit 200 and gave a correction and "nothing happened," although it may not have brought her back down to 100 mg/dL, it might have also stopped her from hitting 300 (which is where she'd have gone in the absence of the correction). In the same situation with different variables (like a different meal with fewer proteins or fats), she might have given the second correction and plummeted to a low blood sugar (especially if she was extra active that day, forcing her into a more "insulin sensitive" state from level one blood sugar impacts).

In order to master diabetes, you need to look at the whole picture, and until you do, you're stuck in a reactive experimentation mode. So, as you build out your understanding of what the three levels of blood sugar impact are currently doing to your blood sugars (*past*, *present*, and *predicted*), it's important to map out strategies that keep you in range at healthier blood sugar numbers for longer periods of time without ending up in the hospital. Be careful, and stay curious. And like the rest of us "Renegade Warriors," you'll benefit more if you continue to *think differently.*

In Chapter 8, I'll walk you through something that's so different, it might just blow your mind (I'll even share how I discovered blood sugar formulas in the first place, and how you can too).

Notes:

_____

_____

_____

_____

_____

_____

_____

_____

_____

_____

_____

_____

_____

_____

_____

_____

CHAPTER 8

INDEPENDENT TIMELINES

Growing up, my dad taught me to fix everything myself whenever possible (cars, the house, and even appliances or toys). I believe that this skill gave me the vision to see things for what they could be instead of just what they are, especially as related to my diabetes management.

There's this one time from high school that stands out when he had me fix my car, and I had no idea what I was doing. Anytime something went wrong, he would be there to help me, but there were a number of times when the car would make these really weird noises, and I had to start problem-solving for myself. I looked at the engine, wanting to find any and all of the parts that could potentially be causing the sound and just replace everything that might be an issue so that I *knew* it was safe (I also wanted to make sure it was ready for my weekend trip beach camping, so there was extra incentive to be quick about it as well). My dad laughed and explained to me that if we replaced everything all at once, we wouldn't have a clear picture of the root cause or know if it was truly fixed because we would likely only be solving the symptoms.

It's like duct-taping a broken pipe back together. It'll hold for now, but the pipe is still broken, and eventually, it's going to burst again. All in all, we ended up fixing the car. It turns out it was the timing belt, which was really tricky to change out on an older car, but knowing that we got to the root cause of the issue gave me peace of mind and taught me a valuable lesson about life—do it right the first time so that you don't have to come back again and again for the same problem—and it ended up saving me quite a bit of money as well (not having to buy parts that didn't need fixing).

66 ——————————————

In life and with diabetes, it's important to change only one thing at a time until you get to the root cause, to fix or experiment in isolation so that you can figure out what the true cause of the issue is and know if it needs a deeper look.

—————————————— 99

I took this lesson and applied it to my diabetes during my experimentation phase when I recognized that different diets had different impacts on blood sugar, but I also recognized that different combinations of similar foods (even within the same diet) had different effects on blood sugar as well. I could eat the same sandwich every day for lunch, but what would happen if I added a fruit smoothie instead of a salad on the side? What would happen if I changed the type of bread or added extra cheese? As I removed and added single (independent) variables from my meals, the different outcomes became more and more clear. I might have a fruit smoothie for breakfast and add scrambled eggs, and the spike wouldn't be as bad as it was the day before when I had the same carbs, but no eggs. I started recognizing consistent impacts with similar macronutrients (carbs, fats, proteins), where if eggs reduced the spike because they were higher in fat and protein, maybe I could just add a glob of peanut butter to the smoothie itself to achieve a similar outcome (because peanut butter is high in fat as well).

We've been misled into believing that "eggs" or "bread" or other foods are good or bad for diabetics, but that's just because nobody had dug deep enough to see that it wasn't the food, but the *type* of food—the macronutrients that had the actual impact. I started playing with different combinations of foods, diet protocols, and even recipe exchanges and noticed something incredible across the board: it really *is* all about the (macronutrient) numbers. *Everything* started with the macronutrients and the numbers that followed. Numbers gave me more certainty. I could "count on" numbers to deliver consistent results with my blood sugar numbers (more numbers again), so I looked deeper into the numbers behind food and found the "glycemic index" (more numbers) that explained that not all carbohydrates are the same; some are more or less likely to cause a spike in blood sugar depending on the glycemic index (and glycemic load) number. In fact, here's a fun experiment to try: google one of the foods in your next meal and then add "glycemic index" after it (like "banana glycemic index"), and you'll see a rating score between 0-100, where the higher the number, the more likely you are to see a spike in blood sugars as a result if you don't adjust your blood sugar formulas.

Though the discovery was slightly overwhelming, light bulbs were going off in my head at the possibilities that lay in front of me. "Diabetes math" started forming in my head, and I felt like a mad scientist on the verge of a breakthrough. But then I began to recognize that there are so many other variables within diabetes that can also impact the spikes or drops that we see on our graphs other than just food. I might have a meal that's low on the glycemic index (less likely to spike my blood sugar), but if my pre-bolus timing was too short, then I'd still spike. And what if it didn't have anything to do with the food I ate at all? What if I did everything perfectly with my carb counting, my macronutrients, and my pre-bolus, but maybe I was on a new medication, exercise plan, or work schedule (remember our "level one blood sugar impacts" from the previous chapter)? I had more work to do, but at least I had a plan now. If I kept *everything* consistent and only changed one thing, one variable at a time, I could track averages to see if that *one* thing I changed led to a different outcome over a few different attempts (in other words, I'd keep the single change for a few days, like eating a different breakfast, to see if the *average* response was consistent each day - watching for either a rise, drop, or stable blood sugar numbers each time).

For example, if I had worked out earlier in the day (let's say I completed a workout first thing in the morning in a fasted state), the spike from my breakfast would also be reduced because I was more insulin sensitive. But, in the absence of the workout, I was more likely to see a spike because my baseline insulin sensitivity was lower (meaning more insulin resistant that day). So, instead of testing each independent variable every single day, I recognized that if I just kept my day as consistent as possible and changed one variable every couple of days (to allow for multiple attempts at each variable, from which I could take an average of the data), I would be able to document consistent patterns and see which variables had the largest overall impact on blood sugar.

As you might already be thinking, yes, this took an incredibly long time. It is wildly unrealistic for most people, and I had to be painstakingly meticulous with my documentation and data analysis—not to mention the constant dance with danger as I experimented on myself without medical oversight, venturing into largely uncharted territory with blood sugar formulas.

Consider this book a consolidation and organization of my findings so that you have a foundation to start with without having to put yourself through that suffering, sacrifice, or sadness.

So, for multiple years, I ate the exact same breakfast, exact same lunch, exact same dinner, completed the exact same workouts, and lived my very own diabetic version of "Groundhog Day" where I would change out one variable at a time to test things to the smallest degree possible in an attempt to remove the mystery from my data. Alongside my personal experiments, I also researched a variety of well-known and trusted sources to confirm or deny my findings. I studied metabolism, exercise physiology, and even psychology to better understand my blood sugars. Sometimes, the answer would be as simple as a single piece of food, like peanut butter toast, added or removed, while on other occasions, it could be something as seemingly far-removed as an emotional swing from an argument I had with someone on the internet.

Other times, I would change the entire diet dramatically—I tried just about all of the fad diets for diabetics (about once every three months, I'd do one *big* blood sugar variable switch in the level one category): LFWFPB vegan, high fat/low carb, high protein, if it fits in your macros (IIFYM), paleo, dirty bulk, borderline keto, you name it—all while keeping my other lifestyle choices consistent to see what changed in respect to my blood sugars. I documented religiously. It started on the back of napkins, receipts, and even on my hand or in my phone notes if I couldn't find anything else to write on. Then I moved to notepads and journals to keep me more organized, and it eventually led me to create what is now called the *Trending Health Journal* (https://trendinghealthjournal.com) that you can buy to this day if you're looking for a simplified and straightforward way to document your blood sugar variables and find patterns. This was my process for experimenting *in isolation* in order to determine the impacts of different diets on blood sugar, as well as to see the impacts of different types of exercises, sleep patterns, stress management strategies, and so on. Time-consuming and obsessive? Yes and yes, but I did it and share it now so that you don't have to.

*****

How Life Impacts Diabetes

See, diabetes, like many other challenges in life, does not exist by itself in a vacuum, unaffected by the outside world. When blood sugar doesn't cooperate, it impacts other areas of our lives, like having to cancel plans with family or friends because of a stubborn high, adjusting (or stopping) workouts because of an urgent low blood sugar, CGM alarms messing with sleep quality, and so much more. But I don't hear anyone else talking about the other side of the equation: how life impacts diabetes. If you remember from our recent chapter, level one blood sugar impacts are the lifestyle habits that can impact our blood sugar responses day to day by manipulating our insulin resistance or insulin sensitivity.

So, take, for example, a sandwich I ate for lunch. I know that I need to take insulin for the carbs in that sandwich, but is it really as simple as taking insulin and enjoying it (like many of us were told on diagnosis day), or is there more to it? Like, what if my insulin sensitivity has improved because of a recent workout or walk? What if the type of sandwich is different from my norm because my favorite shop ran out of turkey and subbed it with roast beef or a different type of bread? We have to pay attention to each independent variable at play, at least in this discovery phase of our diabetes. Different types of foods, types of workouts, subcategories of variables like "type" of carbohydrate and insulin injection location. It can get maddening when you really stop to consider how many different types of impacts there are on blood sugar (slow, medium, and fast impacts as well). Was it something I ate, is it something I'm thinking (such as anxiety increasing heart rate and cortisol production), is it something I'm experiencing (physical pain-causing inflammation and a stress response in my body), and so on?

The good news is that if you remember the last chapter with the three levels of impact, you'll realize that diabetes is all about connecting the dots between interacting blood sugar variables. How does one event, like working out, impact the next event, like a meal? Well, if I worked out, that's a level-one impact if it's in the *past* that will increase insulin sensitivity. I'm about to have a meal, so I need to know what matching my insulin and carbs looks like and how much protein I'm about to eat—that's in the *present* (level two). Secondarily, when outside forces *do* act on our blood sugar, how long do they impact it? What are the timelines of effectiveness? Surely, the sandwich I ate isn't going to spike blood sugar for the next month straight, but it's going to last longer than the moment when I take my last bite as well. It might continue to spike for an hour or two if I make an error as it continues to digest. The workout I had this morning has had a lasting impact on my insulin sensitivity as well, but for how long? A few hours? A few days? It's with the awareness of these external (level one) variables in the past that we build our "blood sugar map" (which may be a future book I write as the topic is far too deep to cover in a single paragraph). If I'm aware that my workout this morning is still impacting my blood sugar at lunch, these "mysterious fluctuations" that lead to frustration and anxiety begin to finally make sense, and I can now anticipate how my strategies must change in order to keep stable and in range blood sugar. This allows us to live our lives with more peace of mind and confidence as the uncertainty and fear melt away.

✴✴✴✴✴

Making Informed Decisions

Understanding how long different timelines are active and impacting blood sugar in our diabetes management decisions allows us to make more informed decisions as we navigate through the chaos. For example, I once heard it said that a high-fat snack can impact blood sugar (technically through insulin resistance) for up to eight hours. So, if I have a snack of eggs and cheese in the late morning (like I did today), I might consider adjusting my insulin dosing strategies for lunch and potentially even dinner as a result of a variable that was introduced in the past. It's kinda like if I felt tired during the day and didn't know why, I might consider something in the now (level two variables), like a workout that could have made me tired, but in the absence of a *present* variable, I begin to look backward, into the *past* (level one), to identify the fact that I didn't sleep well the night before, and *that's* why I'm tired in the present. We're already using many of these methods in our everyday lives, we now need to focus them intentionally towards our diabetes management.

Something that happened in the *past* was impacting my *present,* and it will do so until I balance it out with something of an *equal and opposite* reaction, like coffee or a nap in this example (level two variable). If you think back to "retrospective analysis" from earlier in this book, that's all this is: looking backward with our diabetes detective hats on to find the root source of our difficulty so we know how to fix (or balance) our problem. So much of this "retrospective analysis" method is just us getting curious and looking back at the decisions we made or didn't make that might be impacting our current blood sugar in the now. Following the discovery of what's causing our blood sugar problems, we then, of course, have our level two "balancing arrows" strategy to pick from to determine our best course of action to balance it out and achieve stable blood sugar once again.

Another way to phrase this framework is **"global" versus "local" impact**. If I'm looking for the source of my blood sugar problem right now (in this case, we'll say it's a blood sugar spike), I have to think about the sandwich I just ate ("local" or "small picture" impacts), plus also think about my recent history and the fact that I didn't sleep last night, I skipped my workout this morning, and I went to a barbecue yesterday where I had some really high-fat food (these are all "global" or "big picture" impacts as we zoom out on the situation). All of those impacts are going to affect my blood sugar for the next twenty-four to maybe even seventy-two hours, depending on which of those variables were encountered or combined. By zooming out like this (looking at the "global" or big picture impacts) and then looking backward (retrospective analysis), we can see a lot more of the potential impacts that might be pushing our blood sugar up or down. This gives us context to the blood sugar numbers that we see.

When we think about these independent timelines (like how long *each* variable impacts our blood sugar independently from the others), we have to look at them as solo experiments to be conducted. So, if I want to know the impact of a high-fat snack and see if it truly lasts for eight hours, like I've been told, I'll have to introduce the high-fat snack and have that be the *only* variable that changes. It's just like when my dad told me to replace only one part in the car at a time to then test and see if that was the root cause of the problem. We must test *in isolation*, experiment *in isolation*, and document *in isolation* (like fats in this example) to identify if that's the reason we've been seeing undesirable blood sugar fluctuations (like the delayed rise of blood sugar) or if something else was to blame. The only way we can truly identify the cause of our undesirable blood sugar fluctuations is to test *in isolation*, document, analyze what happened, and assess the graph. This helps us to avoid the classic pitfall of mislabeling the root cause with something that's more tied to correlation instead of causation.

Here's an example from one of my clients on a recent coaching call:

Client: I can't tell if my morning coffee is causing the spike in my blood sugars. How do I know for sure?

Me: Tell me all the details of your morning so we can get more clarity on potential causes first.

Client: I wake up at seven, make my breakfast of oatmeal and a few blueberries with scrambled eggs, and drink my coffee as I sit down to work from home. I see a spike as soon as I get to my first meeting almost every day.

Me: Okay, so a quick recap of things that could possibly lead to a spike in blood sugars: "dawn phenomenon" or feet on the floor as your liver dumps stored glucose into your bloodstream, possible improper basal rates from your insulin pump in the background, incorrect insulin-to-carb ratio for your food, error in carb counts, too short of a pre-bolus (insulin timing), microbiome/gut response to certain foods, stress from sitting down to work, dehydration, dinner from last night if it was high in fat (yes, kinda crazy, I know), and finally, yes, possibly the caffeine from your coffee.

Me again: So is it reasonable to assume that with all of those variables, it's impossible to know with absolute certainty that the coffee is the sole reason for the spike in blood sugars since there are so many other variables at play at that moment?

Client: Okay, yes. But how would I know?

Me: Let's remove the coffee and see if the spike still occurs (how terrible to skip morning coffee, I know), or we can adjust the time that you consume coffee to be either earlier or later so that we can test that *single* variable *in isolation* on a different *timeline* in an attempt to determine whether coffee *by itself* causes a spike. Then, we can create an action plan based on our findings. Sound good?

Client: Makes total sense. Thank you.

Me: Awesome! Alternatively, we could (and should) confirm all other variables as we go (basal rates, insulin-to-carb ratios, etc.) so that there's more certainty overall as well.

Client: Yes, I'd love to know that those are all correct as well. Looking forward to it.

See how that works? This is also why it can be extremely difficult to identify the root cause of crazy blood sugar when life itself is crazy. Chaos begets chaos. If you're able to slow down for a few days to truly observe and intentionally test and document the potential causes of blood sugar ups and downs, it's likely to have a lasting positive impact as you finally discover some clarity in your blood sugar patterns. If you know the problem that you're solving (like my client discovering that it wasn't coffee but actually a pre-bolus timing issue that led to the morning spike each day), you're able to introduce more *flexibility* as a result because you know how to adapt properly to a greater variety of situations. Life gets more fun as a result of the work you put in. Work now, play later.

Note for independent timelines and testing *in isolation*: Consistency wins over all else in an experimental phase. During that time of my life, when I kept everything consistent and only changed one variable at a time, my blood sugar was ridiculously predictable. That being said, I'll be the first to admit that it was not the quality of life I'd like to settle for in the long run because I was eating the same food at the same time every single day: same insulin, same workouts, same bedtime. I was saying no to going out with family and friends. I said no to travel, no to fun. It was not enjoyable or spontaneous, but during that time of my life, I was on a quest for certainty. I needed to know why my blood sugar did what it did. And I got my answer when I tested the different variables one at a time.

What happens if I keep everything consistent but go to bed late?

What happens if I eat all the same foods but skip breakfast one day and try out intermittent fasting?

What happens if I exercise at the same time every day, but this week, my exercises are significantly more intense, longer, or of a different type?

As you can tell, there were a *lot* of experiments and findings, and as my clients often tell me, "Matt experiments so that we don't have to," which is true. My experiments have continued over the years, and my clients have access to an entire video vault where I log my findings to some of the most popular and useful topics like "how to dose insulin for proteins and fats," "insulin adjustments for a night out with alcohol," or my personal favorite, "expectations vs reality: how to enjoy spontaneity without giving up controlled blood sugar."

I obsess over the details so that my clients don't have to. They get a head start that saves them years of frustration, and I hope this book provides you with a similar benefit.

When we change one variable at a time in these testing and experimentation phases, we know that the resulting blood sugar (with relative certainty) is a result of that single variable change.

Now, I also recognize that most of us living with diabetes don't live inside a box where nothing changes day to day, allowing us to maintain a consistent routine forever. And I also recognize that even if you did, as I did for a short period of time in my life, it can be miserable and depressing to devote your life—every single moment of every single day—to identifying blood sugar trends and researching them and analyzing them and trying to determine why blood sugar is not cooperating the way that you want it to. This is why I wrote this book. This is why we have coaching programs. This is why I work with people one-on-one. I realize that you probably don't have multiple years to dedicate twenty-four hours a day of your attention and focus to diabetes in the hopes that you figure it all out; you've got a life to live.

My goal with this book is to share information with you that allows you to shortcut your progress, take my decade-plus of T1D experience and research with experimentation, and implement what I learned while building on top of it for yourself—to "stand on my shoulders" so to speak. If you understand that "**consistency yields consistency**," then you're able to take a few days, weeks, or months to experiment with a few single variables to identify the potential causes of blood sugar that wrecks your day. If you can properly identify the root cause of what's been messing with your blood sugar, you're one step closer to fixing it for good. As we work on building a deeper understanding of independent variables, we get to move on to the next topic, which is to have a look at what happens when we cross more than one variable at a time and see how they impact each other when life does get crazier. Next, we learn how to handle the chaos and adapt our strategies for more spontaneity.

PS: If you remember, in the previous chapter, we talked about "**balancing arrows**" (your level two impacts and actions), where experimenting to determine your independent timelines and identifying which of the variables cause blood sugar to go up or down is actually your process of mapping out your toolbox of "**balancing arrows.**" So if, while isolation testing, you recognize that rice makes your blood sugar go double arrows up, but oatmeal is only slanted up, this is what it looks like for you to build out an understanding of how your body works and understand which tools you have available to you as you manipulate your blood sugar using the "balancing arrows" framework. A walk is a slow drop, but running is a fast drop. Great, now which *types* of foods would best balance that out? Test *in isolation*, document and analyze your findings, and implement your action plan. This is the "**Renegade Warrior**" way.

My client, who wanted to test coffee *in isolation* to see if it was the reason for the spike after breakfast, might have identified that the root cause for the spike was actually the pre-bolus timing, but they *also* noticed that coffee does require insulin when consumed *in isolation* as well. She's effectively added a new variable to her "**balancing arrows**" checklist. Now, if she's got a dropping blood sugar but hasn't had her coffee yet, she knows that even black coffee will lead to a blood sugar rise and can be used in place of sugar if no sugar is available (or desired). The more options you have, the more adaptable you can be in life. The more adaptable you can be, the easier it is to live your life on your terms without giving up controlled, stable blood sugar.

In our program, we like to use the acronym **CANI (Constant And Never-Ending Improvement)** as a way of life. The day you stop learning is the day you start falling behind. Personally, I'm *still* learning about blood sugar and adding new "balancing arrows" options to my toolbelt. The other day, I learned about the blood sugar-lowering impact that heavy study or thinking can have because the brain uses up glucose when you're deep in thought. How crazy is that? Always learning, always a student.

Notes:

_____

_____

_____

_____

_____

_____

_____

_____

_____

_____

_____

_____

_____

_____

_____

CHAPTER 9

INTERDEPENDENT TIMELINES

With my blood sugar at 90 mg/dL and double arrows down (rapidly falling), I hopped off the treadmill in complete shock, trying to wrap my head around why it had dropped 130 points in such a short period of time. Looking back, I can tell you that I was stacking blood sugar variables with what we now refer to as an "**accelerator**." An "accelerator" is something that makes another variable more efficient or effective in moving blood sugar in one direction or another. For example, if I take insulin and then go for a run (like in the example above from earlier in the book), I'm able to use the run to make the insulin work faster than it otherwise would (increased heart rate, circulation, blood pressure, and so on, in addition to its independent impact of a glucose burn rate as previously discussed). This is neither good nor bad because, depending on the situation, it could be either.

However, by understanding that the timing and volume of my insulin dose can be manipulated based on what I deem helpful (I can delay a dose or even adjust how much I dose), I'm able to further dial in my strategy of pushing blood sugar in the direction I want, when I want. Alternatively, if I recently gave insulin and have the option to go for a run now versus later, I can use my knowledge of the situation to determine whether I would benefit more from a run now (which would accelerate the insulin on board, more beneficial if I'm already at a higher blood sugar and want it to come down) or if I'd benefit more from letting the insulin do its thing first while my food digests before going on a run later (like if my blood sugar was already in a lower zone and I didn't want it to drop further). What's interesting as well is that it's not only limited to insulin and exercise. These "interactions" exist between *all* blood sugar variables; they're just not all as easy to observe as this example of exercise accelerating insulin on board from a recent dose.

In fact, one of the most shocking variables I ran into (by accident) is that if I take a hot shower while I have insulin on board from a recent dose, my blood sugar tends to plummet much faster than it would otherwise. This can be used as a strategy, but it could also catch you off guard if you're unaware of this interaction between variables. Once upon a time, I finished a workout, went directly into taking insulin for a smoothie (that I'd drink right away), and then hopped in the shower to wash off the sweat from the workout. I didn't realize this for years, but I had effectively (and luckily) balanced my blood sugar. The smoothie would have caused a rapid rise in blood sugar in the absence of an appropriate pre-bolus, but the hot shower accelerated the insulin's action, allowing it to catch up to the smoothie, preventing a spike and keeping me stable as a result. For me, getting into a jacuzzi also has the same impact as taking a hot shower.

Building out our deep understanding of these variable interactions is critical if we want to avoid these potentially dangerous pitfalls (like if I took insulin for my smoothie but took the hot shower first *before* drinking the smoothie, I could have ended up in the hospital). In fact, something unique that I need you to understand before we move forward is that when you combine different variables, their independent timelines may be altered as well. That might sound complicated, so what exactly do I mean by that? In isolation, eating carbs before going on a run might lead to stable blood sugars and work quite well. But when those same carbs are consumed alongside fats (like scrambled eggs I had with my banana recently), the fats will slow down the digestion of the banana, altering the timing of blood sugar impact. When I tried the banana alone before my run, my blood sugars were perfect. I had effectively balanced the arrows (up arrow from the banana and down arrow from a run). When I added scrambled eggs to the equation, my blood sugar went low during the run and higher after the run (because of the delayed digestion of the eggs and resulting delayed blood sugar impact, the run had an immediate lowering impact on blood sugar, and the food had a delayed rise impact, leading to an imbalance in the timing).

Knowing this, if I *really* wanted to have the eggs, I need to know *how* the eggs will alter the timing (aka *timeline*) of the impact and might consider having the food earlier so that the new timeline (digestion being slowed because of the fat in the eggs) outcome matches with what I want (which would be a rise in blood sugar at the exact moment that I start my run, not at the end of my run when I no longer need it). Let's look at a visual of what a "standard" morning looks like to get an idea of how these variables are overlapping (the timeline bars beneath the arrow line suggest how long each of these variables remains "active" with their impact on blood sugar levels, ignoring for a moment the actual up or down impact on our blood sugar):

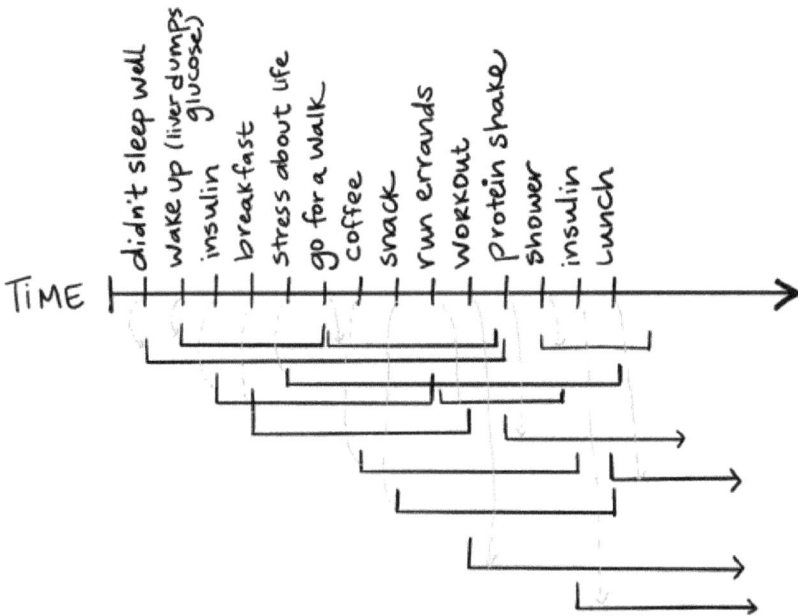

As you can see, *everything* we do has an impact on blood sugar management and often *continues* impacting blood sugar for hours on end. I'll give you another example from a recent Marvel movie franchise that explored this concept called the "multiverse," where the theory states that there isn't just *one* Earth, but rather an infinite amount of different versions of Earth that exist throughout all of space and time. If you don't follow, just stick with me, and I'll do my best to simplify this. In the "multiverse" theory, there are an infinite amount of universes, and they all exist concurrently (at the same time). In each of these different universes, there are different realities, sometimes vastly different from each other, and sometimes having only slight differences. So, for example, if we have the superhero Spider-Man[2] in our universe, you might find in a different universe that they have a superhero called Beetle-Man, and in a third universe, he might be just a normal guy with no superpowers at all.

In your normal day-to-day life, your blood sugar may respond relatively consistently because you're not changing any of the interacting variables (we are creatures of habit, after all). But when you change up your routines with travel, weekend experiences, or a date night out, it's like traveling to a different universe where the rules of blood sugar are a little different. Sometimes, it's only a minor adjustment, like traveling to a destination with just a one-hour time zone difference, but other times, it can feel like entering a whole new world—like when I started training for my Ironman races and had to consume around 400 grams of carbohydrates in a single training session just to avoid going low (though I did stay 100% in range the entire time). Interdimensional travel through the multiverse—aka, living a full and spontaneous life with Type 1 diabetes—*is* possible; you just need to know what to expect (aka, set up your blood sugar formulas) in order to do so safely.

Alternatively, this multiverse example is also like the subtle differences we all experience in our responses to all of the different blood sugar variables

---

[2] Spider-Man is a registered trademark of Marvel Entertainment, LLC.

day to day. I might drop 50 mg/dL when I go for a jog, but maybe you drop 100 mg/dL. Someone else might not drop at all but actually spike. We all have different "realities." We all have diabetes, but it might look different *in our world* than it does for someone else. This is why it's important to look at how *your* blood sugar responds, and it's especially important to recognize that cookie-cutter approaches for diabetes management will not work the same for everyone. This is why **we are "renegade warriors." We** *think differently*. And if you haven't caught on yet, this book doesn't teach generic strategies for diabetes management as much as it teaches you *how to think*, a much more valuable skill set, in my opinion.

When we look at the different "realities" of blood sugars, we also have to consider that different variables might change in different *contexts*—this is where the second half of the "multiverse" theory comes into play. If you've ever watched a movie that had time travel in it, at some point or another, they usually say something like, "Don't touch anything in the past. It'll mess up the future." With our blood sugars, if we are constantly changing out variables while testing and experimenting, it's sure to change the way that those variables interact, and it's also going to change how those variables respond (which might be different than we're used to).

Let's put those two examples together now and try to make some sense out of this with Batman,[3] one of my all-time favorite superheroes. Batman started life as a rich kid whose parents were shot in an alley by a criminal when he was young. This gave him a strong hatred of crime and a desire for justice. If Batman went back in time as an adult (or, in the "multiverse" theory, if he went to a different world) and saved his parents from ever being shot, then he would never have become Batman because he'd never have had that trigger event of seeing his parents die, which in turn gave him a hatred of crime and a desire for justice. By changing *just one* variable in the timeline, he would dramatically alter the entire end result and cause a ripple effect throughout

---

[3] Batman is a registered trademark of DC Comics.

space and time. So it is with our blood sugar variables and timelines. Remove, alter, or add a single variable, and we must be on the lookout for the "ripple effect" down the line (remember the "three levels of blood sugar impact" chapter from before?).

Similarly, if you take a blood sugar variable *in isolation*, let's say you're going for a run without any insulin or any food or any other variables acting on blood sugars. Things will likely behave as they have previously, as expected, so to speak. But what happens when you put it in a situation where you're going for a run with insulin on board, and you've eaten food recently? Well, now all the "rules" have changed because we've changed the interacting timelines. In this example, the introduction of the run might independently lower (burn) blood glucose while simultaneously causing the insulin that was recently given to work faster (because of increased circulation and a higher heart rate) *and* might cause a delay or "pause" in digestion (because the body will prioritize working muscle tissue over digestion if the two are happening at the same time).

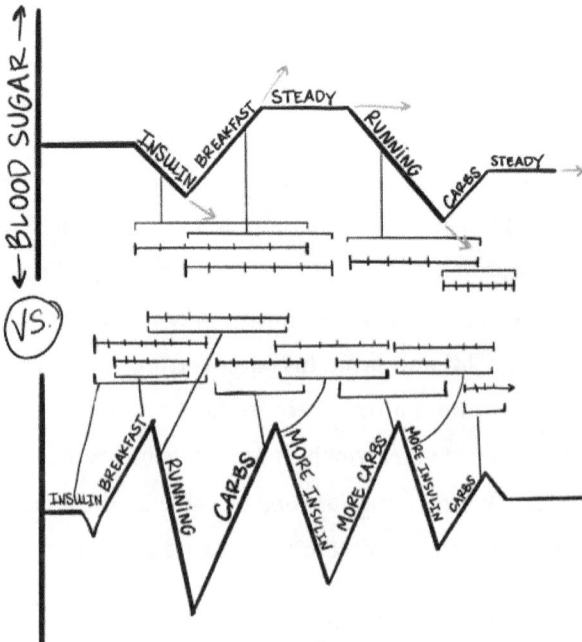

Let's compare these two illustrations. In the top example, we've separated the different variables so that, for the most part, the timelines do not interact and allow for us to view the independent variable impacts (and honestly, make life with type 1 diabetes easier). In the bottom example, we see what happens when we smush the variables together and allow timelines to overlap and interact - absolute chaos.

The presence of a run (our original variable) has effectively shortened the timeline of insulin (made it work faster) *and* extended the timeline of the food (delay in digestion) while also independently burning glucose, which is one of the many reasons this situation leads to a low blood sugar for many of us living with type 1 diabetes. The timelines change as new variables are introduced or removed. So what we have to consider with diabetes is not only what this one variable does every single time I encounter it (like maybe a run leading into a 50-point drop in blood sugars), but rather what this one variable does by itself *in isolation* as an independent timeline, and more importantly (because life with diabetes does not exist by itself in a vacuum void of change), what does this variable do when combined with other variables and how can I expect things to change (so as to proactively adjust and keep blood sugar stable and predictable)?

As you might see in the previous image, the more "spread out" our day is, the easier it is to identify and manage blood sugar fluctuations, as we only have to consider one or two at a time. As our days get more smushed together, the overlapping variables make it more difficult to manage and stabilize blood sugar levels (or even know what the root cause of the fluctuation is).

If I explained that correctly, your mind is blown away with both excitement and curiosity while also being a little (or a lot) overwhelmed by the true complexity of this disease.

Let's break it down as a strategy, using the example above where I went for a run with insulin on board.

So if I expect my run to drop me 50 mg/dL points (which also might change if I go for a short run vs a longer run—food for thought), I have to consider a run combined with the insulin might lead to 50 points dropped from the run, PLUS whatever the expected outcome is from the insulin itself (which would change depending on how much insulin on board were present and how recent the dose was given). Personally, I've experienced an exponential drop in blood sugar when I combine the two (run and insulin), where I get a "bonus" drop in blood sugar when the two are combined. It seems that going for a run helps my insulin "go further" than I anticipated (which is why it can be strategic to exercise without any active insulin on board to minimize the risk of a low in my experience). As I combine different blood sugar variables, I need to be able to calculate and predict where they are going to go based on my knowledge, both of independent and interdependent experiences.

For example, when I want to eat breakfast and then go for a run, and my blood sugar is expected to drop, I need to identify how to adjust my strategy to balance everything out. In this example, I want to run, so that's not changing. What other blood sugar-lowering variables can I play with or alter to balance out the equation? I might consider my insulin and, more specifically, **the *timing* and *volume* of the insulin**. As an intentional calculation, I might consider reducing my pre-bolus timing or reducing the amount of insulin I take for breakfast to avoid the low I expect while running. If I eat my normal breakfast but reduce the insulin I take for it (so that technically, it's not enough insulin to cover that breakfast) and then go for a run, hypothetically, they should all balance out (or cancel out) to a stable and in range blood sugar if I've calculated it correctly. This is because the glucose burn from the run essentially makes up for the missing insulin from breakfast and helps the insulin that I did give to work faster (and sometimes more efficiently).

The easiest way to identify these impacts is, again, to test *in isolation* first. You might have tested and discovered that a run might drop you 50 gm/dL points for every 30 minutes of running (this is a made-up example that I'm using as a reference point—yours is likely different). Now you add in a new variable, like what happens if I add this snack with no insulin during my run (this is what I often do if I typically notice a drop and want to balance that out without making adjustments to insulin). Alternatively, what happens if I add this much insulin (if I typically notice a spike from a run and want to balance that out)? Or even, what happens if I do this run at a different starting blood sugar level or a different time of day completely?

So now it's as if we're creating a mental (or physical if you prefer) chart for each independent variable and all of its correlated interactions with the other variables that might get added in. It's like we're creating a diabetes "spider web of knowledge" or a "Blood Sugar MAP." This allows us to map out the interactions *before* we encounter them so we're better able to predict how to proactively balance our blood sugar with anything we encounter day to day. *This* is how you live life on your terms with type 1 diabetes—intentionally. It's no longer about asking *if* I can have a delicious, carby sandwich, but *how* can I eat a sandwich without the blood sugar spike leading into chaos? When I know what variables are coming my way, and I know how they're going to interact, I'm better able to predict where they're going to go when it happens. What's critical to understand, though, is that some variables have a much larger impact when combined than others.

Let's take a look at a few other examples before moving on. A run plus insulin has a large impact on most. Hot showers plus insulin also have a big impact for most (leading to lower blood sugar coming on faster when combined with higher amounts of insulin on board, in my experience). Food plus insulin has minimal impact if balanced properly (ideally, no impact if we can balance it out with perfect insulin-to-carb, insulin-to-protein, and insulin-to-fat-resistance ratios, and proper pre-bolus timing). This entire concept actually relates back to our "balancing arrows" framework.

As I introduce different combinations of these blood sugar variables, I need to know if all three of them are "arrow down" variables and will lead to a plummeting blood sugar or whether two of them point down and one points up and might lead to a slow drop overall. Getting my "**balancing arrows**" framework set as the foundation allows me to start building out this library in my head of what I expect blood sugar to do based on the independent timelines and reactions, and then we can combine them to map out our interdependent timelines (the "spider web" or "map" of blood sugar). This is what truly unlocks blood sugar freedom. It allows us to see diabetes as a game of balance and not only as a prison of a restrictive and repetitive lifestyle. As we begin to live our lives more spontaneously, we're able to map out the interactions *before* they happen.

*****

Planning Ahead

My sister (who is also a type 1 diabetic) and I went to Six Flags (a roller coaster theme park) not too long ago, and we walked around all day in an effort to get on all of the rides. We both know that walking lowers our blood sugar, and we took that into account upon arrival with temporary basal rate reductions for her and snacks on hand for me (different options that allowed us both to balance out the anticipated drop in blood sugar with different methods).

At lunchtime, we were going to have our food and take our insulin for the food, knowing that the combination of food plus insulin should balance blood sugar (aka our insulin-to-carb ratio). But with the introduction of a third variable, the constant walking around the theme park all day, potentially causing insulin to work faster (and lower blood sugar simultaneously and independently), we knew that the outcome would be different than it is on a standard day at home. So, with walking around a theme park all day added to our "diabetes math" equation, we knew that an anticipated down arrow from walking should be thought of as part of our strategy, and we reduced the amount of insulin that was given for our food to balance the arrows. Because walking drops blood sugar, insulin drops blood sugar, and food raises blood sugar, we reduced the amount of insulin taken to balance the equation and make it more stable.

Alternatively, we could have also eaten more food or stopped walking and sat down for a few hours while the insulin on board ran its course (but that's no fun to wait when there are roller coasters to ride). Looking at different variables and the impacts they have when combined can help us build out strategies to manipulate blood sugar that is too low or too high for our liking. Case in point: she took less insulin, ate with zero pre-bolus, and ran off to catch an event on the other side of the park that I wasn't interested in. She balanced out the lack of pre-bolus because of the immediate activity of walking that sped up the insulin (accelerators).

On the other hand, I had no interest in the show she wanted to see, so I took less insulin but gave a longer pre-bolus while I read a book I brought as I waited for her. I knew that as soon as she came back, we'd be running around again, so I knew that I needed *less* insulin overall, but I also knew that I'd be waiting for about an hour and didn't want to run high for the hour I was waiting, so I optimized for a lower blood sugar in the waiting period by adjusting the *timing* of my insulin pre-bolus in addition to the bigger picture strategy of adjusting the volume of insulin given (total dose). I stayed perfectly balanced while eating without spiking to a high blood sugar, and sure enough, just as she came back after her show, my blood sugar had started to rise (because I didn't take enough insulin for the whole meal, knowing that we'd be walking again soon) and the activity from walking brought me promptly back down to stable blood sugar at around 90 mg/dL.

Note: It doesn't always work out that perfectly. If she were late or early in arriving back to my area, the plan would have to be adjusted… no biggie.

GOLDEN NUGGET #1: Timing and volume are everything. If I had planned to read my book for the next three hours after eating, I'd likely not have reduced my insulin *at all*. Why? Because fast-acting insulin would have done its work and been mostly out of my system by then.

GOLDEN NUGGET #2: Here's my "high-level" decision-making matrix for activity after a meal (taking insulin on board into consideration):

1. **Red Light:** Activity occurring less than one hour since my most recent insulin dose. I will likely see a massive and rapid drop in blood sugar if I am active during this window of time, and action is likely needed to prepare for and adapt to this. Either make an adjustment in the dosing plan, treatment plan, or avoid activity in this time frame if possible.

2. **Yellow Light:** Activity occurring within the second-hour range since my most recent insulin dose. I will likely see *some* impact on blood sugar in this time frame if I choose to be active, so it's good to have sugar on hand and keep an eye on my levels, but I'll probably be alright.

3. **Green Light:** Activity occurring at three hours or more after my most recent insulin dose—I'm basically in the clear to freely have fun. I'll still bring sugar, but the insulin on board is likely low enough that it shouldn't cause a massive disruption. (This is typically when I begin my workouts or training whenever possible to reduce the variability of blood sugars during exercise.)

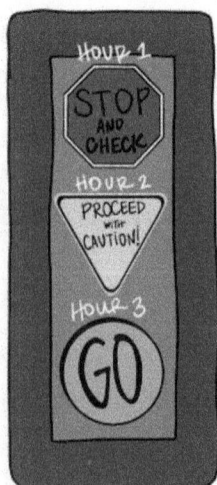

Now, after reading all of this, you might be thinking, *What if I have high blood sugar; can I just not take insulin and go work out because of the anticipated drop if I were to exercise?* Yes and no. It's true that I sometimes drink a lot of water because hydration can assist with any insulin that's given. I then take insulin that I think is appropriate for the situation, and then I might consider going for a walk. Those are three activities that will bring my blood sugar down, and they allow me to do so faster. But if it's not an absurdly high blood sugar (for me, I'd consider something like 160 mg/dL to fall under this category), I might be able to drink water and go for a walk or run without the added correction insulin dose being necessary to bring blood sugar down to a healthier range (*context* is critical though; take insulin when you need it, using exercise exclusively without appropriate insulin can lead into DKA, or "Diabetic Ketoacidosis," which can be life-threatening). If I *were* to add insulin in that example, the water and the walk would accelerate the action timing of the insulin (help it work faster). This is why we call them "accelerators" because they accelerate the action of the blood sugar variable. The last thing I'll touch on in this chapter is the timelines themselves.

Please understand that if I were to take insulin, eat food, and then go for a run without a plan and all within 30 minutes of each other, it would spell disaster for me, and I would likely have a resulting low or high blood sugar (because that's a difficult combo for anyone to master; overlapping variables is trickier than taking on one at a time). However, if I took insulin and waited 20 minutes (my personal pre-bolus timing), ate my food slowly, waited three hours to let it digest and let the insulin run its course, and only *then* went for a run—the entire equation remains balanced because of the timing *between* the variables, and I'd stay relatively stable and in range the entire time (also assuming that I make an adjustment in either carbs or insulin for the run itself - in my case, I consume extra carbs to balance out the drop from running). I've given them time to run their course independently without forcing overlap between the variables. This is the most straightforward path to simplifying your diabetes—spread out the variables as much as possible to avoid overlap (though "simple" doesn't always mean best or even realistic for most of us). Let's revisit the illustration from earlier to drive this point home:

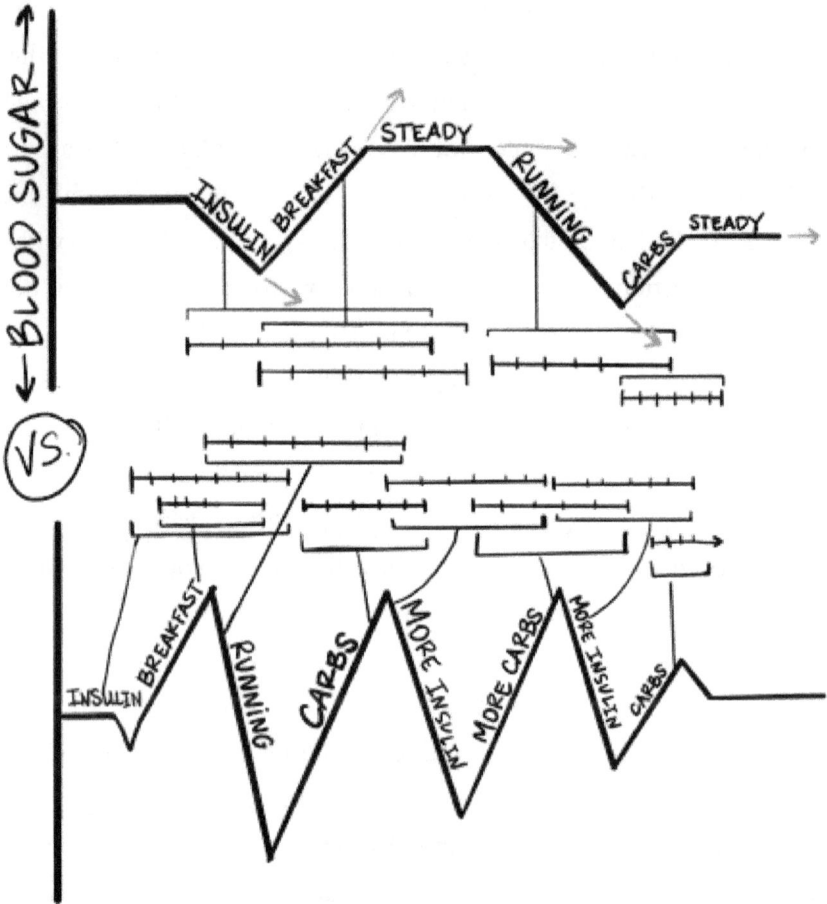

Giving my insulin that 20-minute head start allows it to have time to start working before I introduce my food (this timing *will* likely look different for you, and we cover the exact calculation for determining your down-to-the-minute pre-bolus and other timelines in our programs outside of this book. This is largely influenced by the *type* of food that you eat but also by lifestyle, exercise, insulin on board, and so on). I then eat my food and choose to delay exercise by three hours to wait out all of the insulin on board and give the food time to digest so that when I do finally go for a run, it's in a "timeline" of its own (independent timeline). The more I squish variables together and force overlap, the more that these timelines interact and get muddied (as shown in the bottom half of the image), the more chaotic blood sugars can be, and the more difficult they are to predict. When I live my life in a more consistent routine, I'm able to add and subtract different variables without much thought, but on days when I have a lot of spontaneity with my daughter or when I'm running around on travel days to deliver keynote presentations at type 1 diabetes conferences, it's inherently more difficult to manage blood sugar. This is largely because we can't keep all these different timelines in our heads and at the top of our minds all day long and still have a high quality of life. This is why blood sugar formulas were created, to lighten the load for us "renegade warriors."

With that in mind, I want you to consider two different things:

1. How can I set myself up for success on days when I don't have a lot of responsibilities on the calendar? For example, if I want to go for a 10-mile run (or a 15-minute slow walk, you do what's best for you), I'm probably not going to do it right after I take insulin for breakfast if I have a slow morning with flexible scheduling. I might do it *before* I take insulin and eat breakfast so that it doesn't push me into low blood sugar with all of that insulin on board, and then eat breakfast after I've done my exercise. Alternatively, if I wake up hungry, I might eat and then wait a couple of hours before doing my exercise when there's less insulin on board.

2. The second thing is that the more of these interdependent timelines I'm aware of and have mapped out for myself, the easier, more predictable, and more certain diabetes management gets when I do have busier days with more variables at play. If I can master the interaction of insulin *timing* with other variables, I can master the blood sugar game and fix any undesirable blood sugar with my "balancing arrows" equation. If I know how each of my variables will

interact and am fully aware of all variables that could possibly impact blood sugar, then hypothetically, I could achieve greater blood sugar control than even a non-diabetic (because they see fluctuations in blood sugar day to day as well, but can't really do much about that since their pancreas is the one in control).

I give you this framework as a foundation to build on top of so that you can be aware of other variables that might be impacting blood sugar behind the scenes. So when you take insulin for your sandwich, and it doesn't stay perfectly stable, now you're more aware and know it might be because of something that your doctor never told you about, and not just that "carbs are the devil." You now hold the keys to unlocking a future with blood sugar that is stable and healthy and will allow you to finally have freedom with type 1 diabetes.

In the final chapter, I'll take you through one of the greatest diabetes lessons I've learned the hard way, show you how you can organize the complexity of everything in this book into a simple "roadmap to success," and give you your next steps as you embark on this journey while living your best life with type 1 diabetes.

Notes:

CHAPTER 10

MAP IT OUT

E ver since I can remember, my family has visited the mountains a few times every year to snowboard. A tradition we had whenever coming back from snow trips to Big Bear, CA, was to stop at either Rubio's or In-N-Out, easily two of our favorite places to eat. If you're unfamiliar with it, Rubio's is a Mexican food restaurant, and In-N-Out is a classic American burger joint. Both got their start in Southern California.

This one particular year, I was completely new to type 1 diabetes and was still trying to figure it all out. We decided to stop at Rubio's with the family. My usual order was a chicken burrito special, one of my favorite foods of all time. It's got chicken (obviously), citrus rice, black beans, guacamole, salsa fresca, creamy chipotle sauce, and romaine lettuce, all wrapped in a soft but sturdy burrito tortilla served with a side of chips. I was feeling adventurous this time, though, and thought I'd go with the fish taco plate. Since this was a new food choice for me, I had never carb-counted it before, nor did I even really know what it came with. I had heard through my diabetes educator that you could ask restaurants for their nutritional facts menu and that it was required by law to keep this somewhere on location for chain establishments.

Sure enough, they had a giant menu with calories, carb counts, and more that I could search through. Sifting through the menu, I finally found the fish taco plate and saw that it was a larger amount of carbs than I anticipated (and more than I'd ever eaten or taken insulin for in one sitting). I didn't second guess it as it was printed on an official document from the restaurant itself. I was famished from an action-packed couple of days of snowboarding in the mountains, so I took the insulin required for the food and enjoyed one of the best plates of fish tacos I've ever had.

After eating, we hopped in the car to drive the remaining two hours back home to San Diego, but about five minutes into the drive, right as we entered the freeway, my heart sank, and my face went pale. My parents heard a very concerned and slightly panicked voice in the backseat of the car say, "Mom? Dad?" They heard my voice quivering and looked back with concern. I looked up from my phone calculator and said, "I think I took too much insulin for that meal." They asked what I meant by that, and I said, "I think I dosed for the family platter and not the single-serve plate I ordered…" My dad, thinking fast, peeled off the freeway and doubled back to Rubio's as fast as he could, determined to get me back to a familiar source of food. My parents got me to the front of the line, politely pushing me ahead of people as I was already starting to feel the symptoms of an urgent low blood sugar coming on. Slightly terrified but ready to do whatever it took, we looked at the menu to find the highest carb item we could think of because, as it turns out, I took three times the amount of insulin than was necessary, and I was in danger.

See, I had ended up dosing for 330 grams of carbohydrates, which at that time, with a 1:10 insulin-to-carb ratio, meant I took 33 units of insulin, the largest dose I've ever taken in my life while living with diabetes (and still my largest dose to this very day). I looked at the menu, and I knew that burritos had a lot of carbs, so I ordered my favorite, a chicken burrito special. My parents insisted that I get a side of chips and whatever else was necessary to keep me from going into a further low blood sugar. "Just eat everything you can." I ate that burrito like my life depended on it because, technically, it did. This was my second *full* meal within thirty minutes, and while I was sick to my stomach after force-feeding a full day's worth of food down my throat, color finally began to return to my face.

My parents looked on nervously, asking how I felt because we didn't have CGMs at that time. All I had was a finger-pricking device, also known as a glucometer, to check my blood sugar levels. Over time, my blood sugar did come back up, and I was fine—on the surface. But for the first time since diagnosis, diabetes had shown that it does, in fact, need to be taken seriously and that all it takes is one slipup to end up in a pretty scary (and potentially fatal) situation.

We did make it home safely, but the moral of that story is that, at that time, because I was newly diagnosed, I was missing information that was critical for my survival, and it almost cost me severely. There were gaps in my strategy, and I was ignorant. The tough truth for all of us (even for me today) is that we don't know what we don't know. And the only two ways that I'm aware of revealing what I don't know is to either learn from my own mistakes (as above) or to learn from the mistakes of others (mentors, books, coaching, and so on). I didn't know that there was a simple solution to that scary situation. I knew that a burrito had a lot of carbs and went straight for the only answer I had at that time.

What I didn't know then is that a burrito also has a lot of fat and protein, which means it's going to be slower to digest. And if it's slower digesting, it's probably not the best option for rapidly dropping blood sugar. The drop in blood sugar I experienced could have been a disaster and landed me in the hospital if I hadn't been lucky that day. Instead—and as you're reading this, I'm sure you've put the pieces together—I could have simply ordered and sipped on a soda, and because it's pure sugar, it would have impacted my blood sugar nearly instantaneously. I would have felt fine a lot earlier, and it would have been the smarter choice overall, but I didn't know that yet. I was blissfully unaware, ignorant even.

There are things even now that I don't know (and that you don't know) that may very well one day be learned through severe error. It is for this reason that I hire coaches and mentors at any opportunity to help me avoid learning lessons the hard way and allow me to learn directly from them instead. It's like a shortcut in life that's also customized to your needs. Of course, now, when looking back on that day at Rubio's, everything seems clearer (and oh, so obvious). Hindsight is 20/20, but we don't always get the opportunity to look back. That day, my ignorance could have cost me my life. That's also why, for the first part of this chapter, I want you to understand that "retrospective analysis" is your key to learning from *your* mistakes, but it's also critical to map it out as you go. Take excellent notes. Adjust strategies as necessary. Plot your course. One day, the stars may even align, and we may work together in some capacity, and that is how you learn from *my* mistakes (and skip to the good part).

*****

The Blood Sugar Map

As we mentioned earlier in Chapter 5, looking back at your last 24 hours to identify the problem areas in your graphs is going to help you to identify what can be changed and what might warrant looking further into in an effort to give us a better chance at a smoother tomorrow. Looking back at that situation at Rubio's, I learned pretty quickly from that lesson that burritos were not a good option for treating low blood sugar. They take forever, and they make it nearly impossible to continue eating because they're so filling. But when we look at "**retrospective analysis**" as a strategy to protect us from ignorance, it becomes clear that it's the only path forward if we expect to learn from our mistakes and not wait on our doctors to hopefully give us the answers. "**Retrospective analysis**" gives us a chance to expand our "**blood sugar map**." When we're first diagnosed with type 1 diabetes, it's like we're given a map on day one, just like the old road maps we were given many years ago when I first started driving. Of course, now we have cell phones and cars that give you directions, but there's part of me that misses plotting the course for road trips on real paper.

Back in the day—and I suppose I'm dating myself now—we had to have physical road maps that had a key and legend to decipher landmarks, pit stops, and dangerous areas. We'd see lines from the top to the bottom and left to right overlaid across the actual freeways, streets, and paths to tell us where we were going and how to get there safely. When you're diagnosed with diabetes, it's like you're handed a roadmap, but only one corner of the map is drawn out and labeled. They give you your "neighborhood" directions about how to get around with an insulin-to-carb ratio (which is actually just their "best guess" because they *don't know* how much insulin you need yet; everything is an experiment from the start). They don't even tell you how to get to the freeways or the fun destinations on the map (like how to enjoy more difficult meals like pizza or how to exercise without the blood sugar roller coaster).

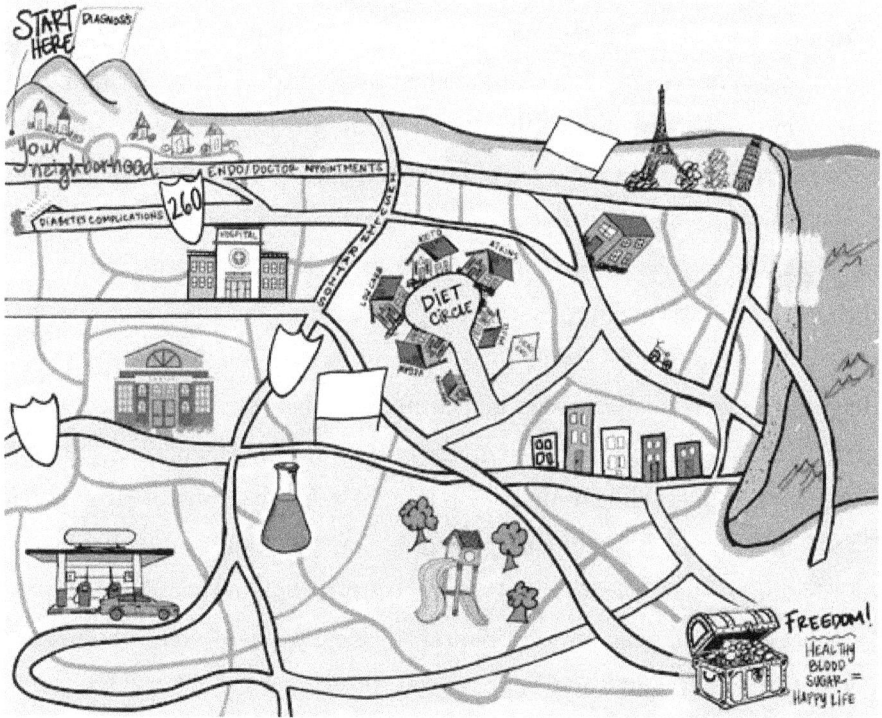

This first step on diagnosis day of them handing you an incomplete map is your medical team's "best guess" at what they hope is the right amount of insulin for you, which is also why they tell you to let them know how it goes (it was a terrifying realization for me that my doctor and endo weren't the all-knowing wizards of diabetes management that I initially thought they were). You were also probably taught that insulin doesn't work instantaneously, and you might need to take it a few minutes before your first bite. You were hopefully taught the basics of how to treat low blood sugar, i.e., **the rule of 15**—eat 15 grams of carbs every 15 minutes until your blood sugar is above 70 mg/dL.

The issue is that that's often all of the instruction that we get. That's all of the guidance. That's all of the map you will ever see from your medical team. This is why "retrospective analysis" is our first step and was born from necessity in my own life. We need to become more aware of what's making blood sugar go up and down so that we *can* start mapping out our diabetes. When I recognized that my medical team was there to help me *survive* but didn't match my goal to *thrive* with diabetes, I needed to figure out what they were supposed to be doing (the "gap" in the medical industry) and then become an expert at it so that I could master my diabetes and live my best life.

Ultimately, "retrospective analysis" allows me to look at my blood sugar and identify what went wrong. This is a great way to expand the map of diabetes that I was given to start seeing the "roads" and the "freeways" and different options on the map to get to my destination. When we're first diagnosed, we're given the road map with that small corner pre-filled by our medical team, and we're told that on the other side of the map, across the vast blank slate in the middle, is an ideal A1C under 7, and a time in range above 70% (both of which should be milestones on your journey, *not* the final destination; I believe we need to hold ourselves to a higher standard).

They tell you what the destination is, "Hey, we need you to be healthy and get your A1C down and improve your time in range." They'll tell you to take care of yourself, but they don't tell you how to get there. There are no actual directions handed to you. They also don't tell you about all the dangerous pitfalls that you might want to avoid (other than the looming "complications" that many of them like to use in an attempt to scare us into action). They also don't tell you about the shortcuts that exist on this map that can make life a lot easier, like our **"balancing arrows"** framework. All they give you is a blank map, and they tell you to figure it out for yourself, try these ratios out, and let us know what you learn works and what doesn't. (You'll see this, along with the treasure chest of Freedom marked on the map previously.) So, "retrospective analysis" is the process of expanding our map based on what we observe to be true for *us* (not the generic "diabetic" in their university books). That's secret number one for how to build your "blood sugar map."

The second phase of this process is that once you have the roads and freeways on the map (just like driving around town and visually mapping out the city, we're "driving around" while we observe our blood sugar with "retrospective analysis" so we can get familiar with how our diabetes works), you need to *label* your blood sugar experiences, assigning meaning to the different blood sugar you see. If I'm experiencing high blood sugar, I can take insulin or go for a walk to bring it down, but it's not going to help me avoid it in the future unless I know the *root cause* of the high blood sugar (so that I can make an adjustment to avoid it the next time). It's helpful to know *why* your blood sugar is high and *why* your blood sugar is low so you can take action to fix it in the present and begin to build out that toolbox for your "balancing arrows" equation proactively to avoid any undesirable situations in the future.

Understand that the more meaning you can assign to the blood sugar you see, the better equipped you are to balance them out in the end. Similarly, if someone was giving you road trip directions and said, "Go straight, turn right, then hook a left, and you're there," you'd have no idea where to turn if the streets on the map weren't labeled. Alternatively, if you had a "local" (aka, an expert) tell you to "Go down Grand Avenue, take a right on Mission Boulevard, and then left on Law Street," you would know specifically how to get to the destination, which in this case is the beach I grew up surfing at (that's where those directions lead in real life—Pacific Beach, CA). Labels give us specificity that allows us to give (and use) directions effectively.

High blood sugar from adrenaline and high blood sugar from food are *very* different, so they must be labeled on your map. If I have repeated high blood sugar every single morning but can't figure out why it's happening, I'm never going to truly be able to fix it. All I can do is repair it at that moment each day with my "**balancing arrows**." If I want to find the source, I need to begin getting curious about the different pieces of diabetes that cause blood sugar to go up and down. This process can be slightly maddening because when you experiment and try to keep things consistent and eat the same things every single day to try to dial in your insulin-to-carb ratios, you might identify other variables that you didn't know were there. And honestly, it can feel like an endless loop of always finding new things that impact blood sugar, but I promise you, it's well worth it in the end. This is where I aim to "shortcut" my clients' efforts and time spent learning, as I'm able to offer a concrete list of variables to select from, and we can get down to the root cause in a single coaching call instead of the months it used to take me when I was originally on this journey of discovery.

For example, if I eat the same breakfast every single day, you'd think that my blood sugar would eventually be perfect for breakfast because I'd be able to fine-tune how much insulin to give since the food itself isn't changing (it's supposedly in isolation). But the issue is that when we look at our level one impacts, the big picture "levelers" from Chapter 7, we see that there are things like sleep quality and quantity that can impact my insulin resistance and maybe even my "dawn phenomenon" in the morning before breakfast. I see that if I skipped a workout the day before, I'm not as insulin sensitive, which means I'm more insulin resistant as a result (remember it exists on a scale) and might need more insulin for the same breakfast meal I usually have. It's not whether you are or are not insulin resistant; it's a question of how much (and how much that impacts our daily decisions). So, if I'm more insulin resistant heading into breakfast, my blood sugar is going to end up higher. If

I'm not aware of a possible increased need for more insulin to combat it, this will likely drive me mad, as I expected it to go smoothly (and it didn't).

We have to be able to zoom out and see the whole picture if we want to be able to keep blood sugar controlled in the constant flux of life, but zooming out becomes a superpower when the map that you're zooming out on is 100% filled out with labels, landmarks, and paths. Understanding your three levels of impact, especially the "balancing arrows" section of what tools are available to you, allows you to label your "blood sugar map" and assign meaning to the roads you take (or don't take). I might look at a plotted path (like wanting to eat pizza) as an example. I know this road is the "scenic route" (going to take a little longer to deal with, but it's totally worth it), where I get to actually enjoy eating pizza because I have the path (blood sugar strategy) dialed in. Oh, this freeway over here, that's a shortcut, right? I can exercise before I eat the pizza so that I'm more insulin sensitive and less likely to spike. Oh, but if I want to stop in at the family park on the map (dessert), I'll need to stop at this gas station before I do so that I can make it there without getting stranded (take extra insulin at the right time to balance everything out with the fats and proteins). I know that if I have high blood sugar, I can take insulin, drink water, and go for a walk, and it comes down much faster and potentially even farther than if I were to just take insulin and wait—there's another shortcut with our "accelerators." So the more of these options we have, the more meaning we can assign to the blood sugar numbers we experience, and the more certainty we have in our response to that blood sugar, which gives us greater peace of mind in the end as we navigate the wonderfully chaotic world of diabetes. As we fill out more of the map and add labels (like the image below), things start to make more sense.

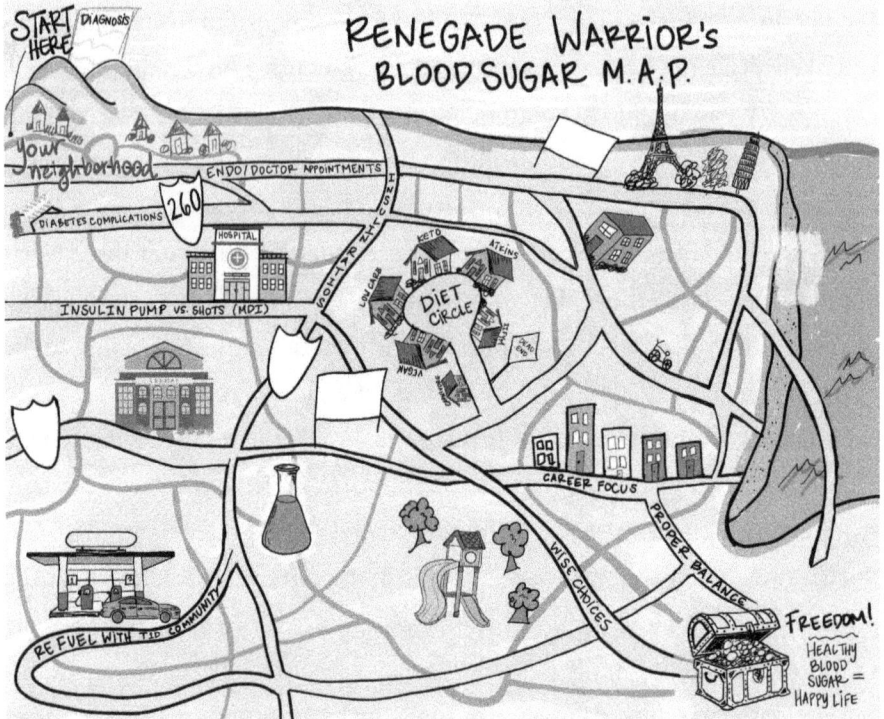

Lastly, to further that second phase of filling out our blood sugar map, we also want to identify the potential pitfalls. I learned the hard way that an insulin correction plus a run can lead to a very dangerous drop in blood sugar and "push" them far lower than I wanted. The more of this map we have labeled, the better we're able to combine desirable blood sugar variables while avoiding combining blood sugar variables that could lead to potential disaster. Our goal in mapping out our blood sugar is to reduce uncertainty and increase the ability to adapt to any given situation.

As we wrap this up, my goal is for you to plot your map and your paths. Once you have the entire map drawn out, with all the signs, streets, and freeways labeled—so you know which paths are the most desirable, which are dangerous, and which are best for you—you can intentionally plot your own course on your terms. This is where something like the personalized macronutrient profiles we teach in my programs comes into play. You hear people all the time talk about which diet is best for diabetics. They'll say that you need to be low-carb, or keto, or vegan, or high-carb, or paleo. The list goes on.

The issue is that they've only mapped out a small section of their map (i.e., the low-carb "neighborhood") and decided that that is the end; that is the goal. They refuse to expand their map because they've found something that works "good enough." And for some people, that's okay. I have no problem with people following a diet that they'll actually stick to if it's working for them. What I don't want people to feel is that they have no option and that they must be restricted to that diet because nothing else is going to work.

The reality is that this "**blood sugar map**" we're drawing out has all of the diets on it. All exercise plans (I'm currently mapping out ultra-endurance training for myself). All lifestyles exist on this map. *Your* map. That's right. Every single diet works for somebody living with diabetes; it just requires a shift in the strategy (the blood sugar formula) being used. The issue is that as you shift between different diets, your strategies have to shift as well. So when we consider low carb, we also need to consider how insulin *timing* and *volume* might change if we ever move to higher carb (even if just for a night out with friends or family).

As we look at keto, we need to understand that a higher fat diet will lead to insulin resistance, and so if we ever wanted to reintroduce carbs, it might be a difficult transition for a couple of days or weeks as our body adjusts and we have to adapt with our strategies (basal and bolus needs *will* likely change). This is not bad, just *different*. I believe that most people don't intend to get locked into a restrictive diet. I believe that most people see a glimmer of hope for the first time when they actually stick to a new diet, and it causes some unhealthy attachment to that diet (sometimes even "cult-ish" attachment in some cases, I'm sure you've seen it online). They think this is as good as it gets and just want to experience more consistency in their blood sugar.

As a result, these people get locked into what they believe is the one and only option for diabetics, but the reality is that if you've got ten people saying they each found a different path that works, and they believe it's the only thing that works, well, somebody's wrong or somebody's lying (or ignorant, as we discussed earlier). So I'm here to tell you that it doesn't matter which diet you pick. All ten people might actually have found something that works well enough for them. But it *does* matter how you strategize with your blood sugars as you build out your blood sugar formulas. Here's the fun part—you get to decide when the map is "full," like the example below, or if you want to keep pushing for more, like me.

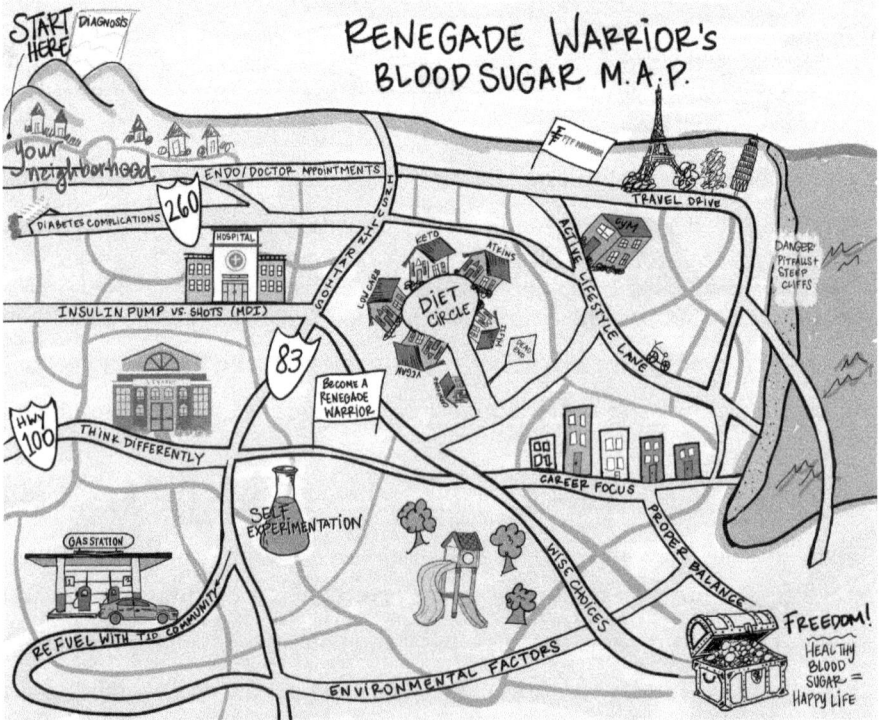

(Note: This "Blood Sugar M.A.P." serves as a visual example, not a complete MAP.)

*****

Becoming a Renegade Warrior

It's important that you find a diet that works for your body and allows you to be healthy with your goals, and then match the right blood sugar strategies to that. You choose the lifestyle, *then* build the strategies for blood sugar to support that choice with balanced numbers. We're not trying to fit our life into the diabetes box - we're going to fit diabetes into our dream life (and that's final). And finally, it must be long-term oriented. If it's a hyper-restrictive diet that you hate, or if it goes against your morals—like an animal rights activist vegan thinking they have to eat meat and low carb to be healthy with diabetes—that's probably not going to work long term because of the cognitive disconnect. What you need to find is one that matches up with your goals and your body's needs. So, when we look at the "**blood sugar map**" as a whole, do you need to be a triathlete like me in order to see stable blood sugar? The answer is no. Endurance sports are just one little speck on the "blood sugar map!" Maybe you're into pickleball or enjoy long walks on the beach. This is *your* blood sugar blueprint.

The reality is that you need to pick what works best for you after you've explored and expanded your maps. I want you to discover first what options are out there, and then we can build the right strategies and formulas for you to live healthy *and* happy.

We build the right path for you depending on what you want to encounter or experience in your life with diabetes. So, if you want the "scenic route," which I would define as the route that has a lot of different food options with spontaneity and adventure, that's fine. It just requires a slightly different strategy than someone who prefers to stay career-focused, be hyper-productive, or be an elite-level athlete. As someone who values more variety, you might have to be ready for the different glycemic indexes you might encounter for different meal types at different restaurants, right? If you want to be an athlete, you have to be ready for the insulin sensitivity shift on hard training days versus rest and recovery days. If you want to be somebody who sits at a desk all day, that's fine, but you have to adapt with your proper strategy and build your map and your path for what works best for you. And this has to be identified and individualized for *you*, which means that you have an active hand in this as well. No more relying on or blaming our doctors and endos—this is *our* life, so we must take responsibility for it. Life with diabetes must be personalized and dynamic at its core if you expect to "have it all."

For me personally, even though I obsessed over blood sugar and researched and experimented, there were still days when I'd be caught off guard, and diabetes would pull me out of the moment, even sometimes completely pulling me away from the task at hand. I needed a way to clearly see what decisions would help or hurt my blood sugar graphs. If I label my map each time I make an error, I can more easily determine which path is the best way forward in the future. That being said, mapping it out takes a lot of time, especially if you're going at this alone. This is not an overnight fix; it's a new lifestyle.

This is the "**renegade way**" that we teach our clients. And we are renegades, or rather "renegade warriors," because **we choose to *think differently***. If you continue to follow the same path that got you to where you are right now, then nothing's going to change, and you'll continue being stuck. But if I *think differently*, if I think outside of the box about what could be, about what I want with life with diabetes, then it allows me to start asking the right questions, like how can I enjoy pizza? How can I compete in a triathlon or an Ironman? How can I be a more present parent or grandparent who makes memories with my children or grandchildren instead of being hyper-focused on blood sugar, or worse, being at the mercy of the blood sugar ups and downs that pull me away from those that I love?

Intentionally filling in and creating our personalized "blood sugar map" brings our strategies together and allows us to build more certainty and peace of mind into diabetes management because we understand how blood sugar works for us. When I went through that near-death experience in Paris mentioned at the beginning of this book, I was mentally wrecked because I didn't have certainty. It's because I didn't know how low my blood sugar levels were going to go that led me to be so fearful of that drop. I didn't know if they were going to come up. And when they did come up, I didn't know how high they were going to go or if they'd plummet back down to another urgent low. It was this uncertainty that led me into madness where I didn't know if things were going to work out, ever. I didn't know if a meal was going to give me stable blood sugar or if I'd go off the charts. I didn't know if a workout would lead me into another low blood sugar or if "this one" would be okay. I was just waiting for the next time things didn't go according to plan. I was always hyper-aware and vigilant (anxious, honestly), and it was exhausting and stole my peace of mind.

So when I finally was able to identify what made blood sugar go up and down as I "labeled" my map, as I discovered how to have more certainty behind balancing those numbers out, it gave me my peace of mind back and resulted in my quality of life increasing dramatically, not only for me but also for those that I love.

An example that I'll share from my own "blood sugar map" is pizza, as this is a really common struggle for most people living with diabetes. Pizza is difficult for a number of reasons, but one of the biggest ones is that it's high carb *and* high fat. Most people living with diabetes either follow a low-carb (high-fat) diet or a low-fat (high-carb) diet. Most of the time, you don't combine the two. Admittedly, it's more difficult to follow a high-carb and high-fat diet as digestion delays are more unpredictable and complicated (though I do tend to follow a similar diet sometimes because I've mapped it out and, ultimately, because I want to enjoy these types of foods). This is one of those "scenic route" options I was referring to earlier, where the strategies required to have stable blood sugar with pizza don't match what's been taught by our medical systems.

It's often why strategies are a rare find for fun foods, like pizza, burgers and fries, milkshakes, or really anything that's a special occasion type of food. With pizza, we have to think of it a little bit differently, like a "**renegade warrior**" would. When eating pizza, I might consider a higher dose of insulin with the higher carb, but I also have to consider how fat might delay the digestion of carbohydrates and, as a result, lead to a blood sugar spike later. Depending on the pizza style, I might also need to count my proteins for a delayed dose (protein converts to glucose over a longer time horizon). The higher fat will delay the digestion of the carbs, but it *also* leads to insulin resistance when consumed in larger amounts.

GOLDEN NUGGET: Fats and proteins can be helpful to delay a spike from carbs, but only to a certain degree, at which point you're essentially "borrowing" stable blood sugar from the future for the "now." In my experience, the higher the fats and proteins are in a given meal, the more stable I am *at first*, but the more difficult and stubborn my high blood sugar is later. Balance is key.

Now, the timelines of these foods and the speed of digestion are what must be mastered if I expect to have stable blood sugar when consuming something like pizza. When I eat carbs, I know that they spike blood sugar, so I do need some insulin up front. When I consume fat, I know it slows down the carbs because the interaction between those two variables *changes the outcome* (revisit the interdependent timelines chapter if needed). So now I know that because it's high carb and high fat, it will impact blood sugar a lot, but it might not all happen right away. I'll have to adjust my insulin timing and might think about a different pre-bolus timing. I might consider an extended bolus if I'm on an insulin pump. I might consider a second (and maybe a third) bolus of insulin to take care of the delayed rise that I see from the higher fat and higher carb combination (especially if on MDI—multiple daily injections).

Where this gets tricky is that with all the different diets that are out there these days, there are different types of pizzas. So now there are low-carb pizzas that are high fat and high protein. There are also high-carb pizzas that have virtually no fat and are largely protein-based. So it's not a matter of generalization on how I dose for pizza. It's how I do it for *this* pizza based on what I know about *my* body's reactions to the different combinations of variables that are present (my "**blood sugar map**"). And ultimately, trying new things is how you master your blood sugar and complete your "blood sugar map." You'll never know how to dose for pizza if you never try because you'll never have the data needed to assess. The first time I tried to master pizza, I went low first (because I took all the insulin up front and the fat delayed the carbs too much, allowing the insulin to "hit" first), followed by a stubborn high later (delayed from the fats and proteins... and the glucose I had to take to fix the initial low). Lesson learned, notes taken, try again with a new strategy.

You need to realize that your strategies will change slightly based on *your* existing lifestyle choices. If you're already used to high fat, then you're likely more concerned with the initial spike from the carbs. If you're already high carb, you're eyeing that delayed spike like a dog staring down a cat about to chase it through an alley. If you're overweight, your body will metabolize that food very differently than an Olympic athlete's body might.

Once again, it's helpful to have a generic strategy going into it, but you need to identify and fill out *your* "**blood sugar map**" if you want precision and predictability with *your* blood sugar.

Let's take one last look at these generic approaches.

What most doctors won't tell you is that you get to decide what your "blood sugar map" destination looks like. They've given you a general cookie-cutter approach of an A1C under 7 and a time in range target of 70%, but I like to hold myself to a higher standard, and I get the feeling that you do too, since you're reading this book and you've made it this far. See, the standards that I hold myself to—that most of my clients hold themselves to—don't match up with what a typical diabetic is meant to experience as an outcome because most people don't think it's possible. But because you're here, as a "renegade warrior," you're utilizing the proper strategies that will allow you to shoot for the stars.

In choosing our destination, we can decide if we want to aim for an A1C that might be under 6, or in some cases with some clients I've seen, even under a 5 A1C with "non-diabetic" numbers. 100% time in range is possible. My average time in range (70-180 mg/dL) over the course of the last five years has consistently been above 90%—all while living my life to the fullest (training for this Ironman, being a husband and a father, owning a business, traveling, eating whatever food I want, you name it).

Now, of course, I have an unfair advantage. I use something called the **"80/20 Blood Sugar Formula,"** as I first mentioned in Chapter 4, *in addition* to everything that I've taught you here. This book was my attempt to cram as much as I could into ten chapters so that you could build the foundation of a successful life with diabetes (not just on paper for your doctor, but one that *you* deem as successful because you actually enjoy it). Using what you've learned here *will* dramatically change your life for the better if used properly and consistently (as a **"renegade warrio**r" would), but the reality is that there is so much more to learn, and much of it must be customized to you. When we consider our unique **"blood sugar map,"** we need to remember that it's not just four or five variables with food, exercise, sleep, and insulin.

There are over 50 variables that impact blood sugar. And each of those variables' behaviors can change depending on what *other* variables are present at that moment in combination with each other (interdependent timelines). So it's no wonder that blood sugar is so difficult to control and why you might have had difficulty up until this point. There are a thousand things going on at once, making it extremely difficult to identify *why* blood sugar seems to differ from day to day and minute to minute (if you don't know what to look for).

In fact, I often encounter two different types of people on phone calls and consults. The first one doesn't know *how* to map out their blood sugars and get these things to a place where they are consistent, predictable, and in control. They have a hard time identifying the exact blueprint to get everything organized and in line so that their blood sugar actually *makes sense*, and they are largely looking for more certainty with blood sugar so they can have more peace of mind and a sense of control.

The second type of person I often encounter on consultations might have been able to "force" controlled blood sugars through restriction, consistency, and sheer determination to make it work, but they're exhausted and frustrated. They've put in so much effort that they don't know if it's worth it anymore, and they want something a bit more automatic (like a formula to lean on). Many times, this second type of person is looking for more freedom and flexibility with their diabetes without giving up the control they worked so hard to achieve. They'd like to use a system that allows for more predictable blood sugar *while they live their lives to the fullest*. This is often a quest for a higher quality of life.

If you fall into one of those two camps (or both in some cases), the good news is that this book will help you take the first steps to start making strides in the right direction. You are in *exactly* the right place, and I'm happy for you. But I want to warn you that going on this journey alone can be exhausting. I highly recommend you get connected with one of our groups or join one of our programs that will provide you with the support and customization you need in order to truly *thrive* with diabetes and be surrounded by other "**renegade warriors**" like yourself. Whether you choose to work with us directly or just use this book to change your life on your own, I want you to know that it's possible to master your blood sugar, and it's something that has been done by myself and hundreds of clients I've worked with personally, as well as thousands of others in our "renegade warrior" groups. I know it can work for you, too, if you're committed, and I'm excited for your journey ahead.

Full disclosure: while I did go through it by myself, it took me quitting my job and focusing 100% of my effort and time, ignoring friends and family and even my wife for the most part. I'm not proud of that or the unhealthy obsession that it required, but I'm just being real with you. All that, and it still took me over two years of daily experimentation, documentation, and risky trial and error to finally identify the **"80/20 Blood Sugar Formula"** that I use today, which is what we teach our clients who work with me directly. Doing this on your own is possible, but it takes immense effort to push the limits of your "blood sugar map" as far as they can go. You might not be after the full picture like I was, and that's okay.

This book serves as a foundation for you to build on top of to simplify your diabetes in a way that doesn't get in the way of your life. For me, with my blood sugar metrics, this looked like the above 90% time in range that I've maintained consistently or the A1C that I have kept in the high 5s and low 6s for the last decade while pursuing my wildest dreams. I also wanted to be healthy and happy, where I was able to start a family, help others, live my life to the fullest, travel, build relationships, and ultimately thrive with diabetes. And I hope that is the same for you as you set out to reach your highest potential. Thank you for giving me your time and attention, and I truly hope this book and anything we may accomplish together in the future was and is immensely helpful.

Notes:

_____

_____

_____

_____

_____

_____

_____

_____

_____

_____

_____

_____

_____

_____

_____

_____

_____

_____

CONCLUSION

Y ou made it to the end of step one! You finished the book and are now aware of a whole new world of viewing, managing, and mastering blood sugar with type 1 diabetes. You've earned the title "**renegade warrior**," and I'm proud of you. Breaking free of the mold is a tough thing to do, especially in the realm of chronic illness. But now that your mind has been unlocked and introduced to this, you probably also recognize that you can't go back to what you were doing before because it's not in line with what you want (or expect) from life anymore. The good news is that I've got you covered for steps two and beyond since you're one of us now.

The first thing you need to know is where you can find ongoing support and more updated information. We have a podcast called *Pardon My Pancreas* on all listening platforms, with hundreds of episodes filled with stories and education. We have a YouTube channel with well over 500 videos (at the time of writing this book) called "FTF Warrior," and you can search just about any other social media platform under the same name of "FTF Warrior" (Instagram, Facebook, and TikTok, etc.).

The second thing you should do is to get on our email list so that you're up to date on all new findings, training, books, and more.

Sign up for our email list, and then poke around for some other freebies on the site if you see anything helpful. SCAN THE QR CODE:

The last thing to think about is whether we might be a good fit for each other in a more customized environment. Give my team and me a chance to get to know *you* a bit more and deliver more customized recommendations for your unique needs. While working directly with me is often waitlisted because our program has gained popularity over the years after being recommended by medical professionals and large diabetes organizations, we do have a number of team members who are dedicated to helping you achieve your goals while you wait for a spot to open up. If you're curious about resources and what's available, here's an image to give you a visual:

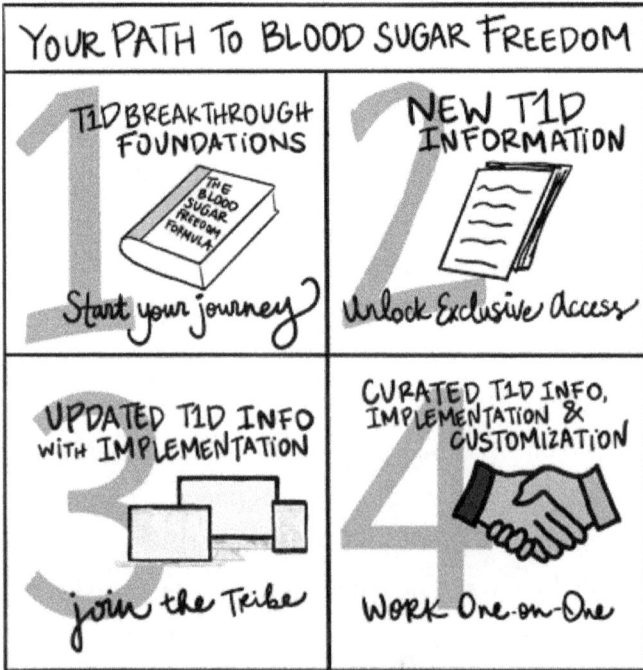

1. Read *The Blood Sugar Freedom Formula* book and take the Challenge to kickstart your transformation.
2. Subscribe to the Renegade Warrior's Newsletter and receive your first issue to enhance your "Blood Sugar M.A.P."
3. Gain cutting-edge knowledge, accountability, and community support with the Warrior's Tribe+
4. Collaborate directly with Coach Matt to personalise your blood sugar blueprint and formulas

Ultimately, my goal is to help you in the best way I can and support you in your efforts moving forward. If we can't find the perfect fit for you, we're always happy to recommend other resources so that you have concrete next steps either way.

It's my hope that you found this book both eye-opening and inspiring. You've now gained diabetes tools and strategies to put in your diabetes toolbox that you can pull out as needed.

You've discovered the "balancing arrows" framework that allows you to bounce back from any blood sugar blunder in real-time.

You've identified those mysterious blood sugar fluctuations with a new understanding of the "three levels of impact" with *past*, *present*, and *predicted* blood sugars, and even how to manipulate your own blood sugar by influencing and adjusting your insulin resistance and insulin sensitivity.

You've seen the importance of learning from your mistakes just as much as your successes in order to map it out (which may become a book in the future; get on our email list to be notified about all things new), as well as plotting your course of action with diabetes management to be one that *you* want and that fits your lifestyle—not one where you have to live under restrictions or be bored to death.

You've watched the whole plan come together with blood sugar formulas as a revolutionary new way to make informed diabetes decisions with more certainty and control in order to maintain more consistency in blood sugar so that you *can* live life to the fullest.

I'm so proud of you and all the effort you've already put into your diabetes management. It's hard work. Diabetes is crazy complicated, and nobody can take this burden from you. Yet, here you are, a "renegade warrior" who stands up in the face of adversity and chooses to keep up the fight.

I'm looking forward to hearing all about your experiences with this book, and I'd be absolutely honored if you left a review online with your honest thoughts on the book now that you've had a chance to absorb all it has to offer (please leave the review on Amazon.com). If you're the kind of person who wants to do good in the world, your review might just be the reason that someone decides to give this book a try and have their life dramatically changed for the better. All it takes is a few minutes of your time, and you could make a difference for someone else who currently is where you used to be: lost, frustrated, and maybe even hopeless with their diabetes. It's by far one of the easiest and fastest ways for you to help us to help more people around the world.

Thank you for your time and consideration, and I look forward to seeing you in one of our groups, programs, or events one day.

Stay strong, "renegade warrior."

And keep up the fight.

THANK YOU FOR READING MY BOOK!

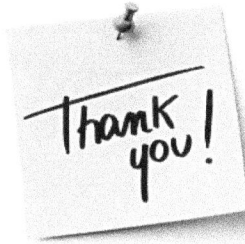

DOWNLOAD YOUR FREE GIFTS

Just to say thanks for buying and reading our book, we would like to give you a few free bonus gifts, no strings attached!

Scan the QR Code:

I appreciate your interest in my book, and value your feedback as it helps me improve future versions of this book. I would appreciate it if you could leave your invaluable review on Amazon.com with your feedback. Thank you!

www.ingramcontent.com/pod-product-compliance
Lightning Source LLC
Chambersburg PA
CBHW031536260326
41914CB00032B/1835/J